"Open this book and accompany an exceptional clinician as she revisits her own evolution with compassion and courageous self-confrontation. Open this book and listen to a superb psychoanalytic mind sharing itself without defensiveness, without idolizing any theoretical gods. Open this book if you are willing to confront your own unformulated assumptions and coax elephants out of their hiding places in *your* office. Open this book to encounter my nominee for World's Most Honest Analyst."

**Sandra Buechler**, *Wiliam Alanson White Institute*

"Joyce Slochower's engaging personal presence suffuses every page of this beautifully written volume. You come away from it with a deeply felt sense of the relational/Winnicottian integration that lies at the heart of Slochower's thinking, and with an appreciation of qualities that are often in short supply: Wisdom, unflinching examination of the analyst's foibles, and—zounds!—humor. Clinicians of every stripe and level of experience will enjoy and learn from *Psychoanalysis and the Unspoken*."

**Donnel B. Stern**, *William Alanson White Institute*

"Joyce Slochower's *Psychoanalysis and the Unspoken* is a self-reflective and affectively connected volume whose immediacy makes you feel as if you are in the room with her. Exploring theoretical and clinical complexities, we see Slochower change and grow over time. The book makes you want Joyce Slochower as a colleague and friend."

**Judy Kantrowitz**, *Boston Psychoanalytic Society & Institute*

"Joyce Slochower's work provides both an accompaniment and a counterpoint to the relational turn. Slochower is known for her important role in challenging and clarifying basic assumptions about clinical theory in relational psychoanalysis. Her thoughtful interpretation and application of Winnicott helps overturn the old paternal bias toward interpretation."

**Jessica Benjamin**, *Beyond Doer and Done To: Recognition Theory, Intersubjectivity and the Third. Routledge 2018.*

"Too few psychoanalytic writers have the ability to skillfully deconstruct and explicate highly complex theoretical and practice issues. Fewer still can accomplish this in clear, concise prose. That Slochower can do both is a rare gift. Nowhere does she manage this feat more elegantly and compellingly than in this newest work, her most important and timely to date. I have no doubt that *Psychoanalysis and the Unspoken* will be a thought provoking and invaluable addition to every clinician's bookshelf."

**Steven Kuchuck**, *DSW, Author of The Relational Revolution in Psychoanalysis and Psychotherapy and Past President of the International Association for Relational Psychoanalysis and Psychotherapy*

"In this brilliant volume, Joyce Slochower skillfully uncovers what we would rather hide, mute or whisper. Fascinating, well-written, and poignant, *Psychoanalysis and the Unspoken* opens our eyes as well as our minds, exploring our secret collusions, illusions, idealizations, and violations."

**Galit Atlas**, *Ph.D. Faculty NYU Posdoc. Author of Emotional Inheritance.*

# Psychoanalysis and the Unspoken

What do therapists not talk about? What do we ignore/miss/sidestep? What factors—personal, social, political—inform our areas of blindness? This book names and explores what psychoanalytic theory often skips over or simplifies—how, when, and why we fail to uphold our professional ideal.

Turning a critical eye on her own theory, Slochower reflects on how it, she, and the field have evolved and what remains unspoken. In so doing, she pushes us to do the same.

With its sharp focus on both theory and clinical work, this book is essential reading for psychoanalysts and psychotherapists.

**Joyce Slochower** Ph.D., ABPP, is Professor Emerita at Hunter College, CUNY; faculty, NYU Postdoctoral Program, Steven Mitchell Center, NTP, Philadelphia Center for Relational Studies & PINC. She is the author of *Holding and Psychoanalysis: A Relational Perspective, Psychoanalytic Collisions*, and is co-editor (with Lew Aron and Sue Grand), of *De-idealizing Relational Theory* and *Decentering Relational Theory*.

PSYCHOANALYSIS IN A NEW KEY BOOK SERIES
DONNEL STERN
Series Editor

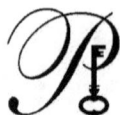

When music is played in a new key, the melody does not change, but the notes that make up the composition do: change in the context of continuity, continuity that perseveres through change. Psychoanalysis in a New Key publishes books that share the aims psychoanalysts have always had, but that approach them differently. The books in the series are not expected to advance any particular theoretical agenda, although to this date most have been written by analysts from the Interpersonal and Relational orientations.

The most important contribution of a psychoanalytic book is the communication of something that nudges the reader's grasp of clinical theory and practice in an unexpected direction. Psychoanalysis in a New Key creates a deliberate focus on innovative and unsettling clinical thinking. Because that kind of thinking is encouraged by exploration of the sometimes surprising contributions to psychoanalysis of ideas and findings from other fields, Psychoanalysis in a New Key particularly encourages interdisciplinary studies. Books in the series have married psychoanalysis with dissociation, trauma theory, sociology, and criminology. The series is open to the consideration of studies examining the relationship between psychoanalysis and any other field—for instance, biology, literary and art criticism, philosophy, systems theory, anthropology, and political theory.

But innovation also takes place within the boundaries of psychoanalysis, and Psychoanalysis in a New Key therefore also presents work that reformulates thought and practice without leaving the precincts of the field. Books in the series focus, for example, on the significance of personal values in psychoanalytic practice, on the complex interrelationship between the analyst's clinical work and personal life, on the consequences for the clinical situation when patient and analyst are from different cultures, and on the need for psychoanalysts to accept the degree to which they knowingly satisfy their own wishes during treatment hours, often to the patient's detriment.

A full list of all titles in this series is available at:
https://www.routledge.com/Psychoanalysis-in-a-New-Key-Book-Series/book-series/LEAPNKBS

# Psychoanalysis and the Unspoken

Joyce Slochower

Routledge
Taylor & Francis Group
LONDON AND NEW YORK

First published 2024
by Routledge
4 Park Square, Milton Park, Abingdon, Oxon OX14 4RN

and by Routledge
605 Third Avenue, New York, NY 10158

*Routledge is an imprint of the Taylor & Francis Group, an informa business*

© 2024 Joyce Slochower

*British Library Cataloguing-in-Publication Data*
A catalogue record for this book is available from the British Library

*Library of Congress Cataloging-in-Publication Data*
A catalog record has been requested for this book

ISBN: 978-1-032-66020-2 (hbk)
ISBN: 978-1-032-69152-7 (pbk)
ISBN: 978-1-032-69153-4 (ebk)

DOI: 10.4324/9781032691534

Typeset in Times New Roman
by Apex CoVantage, LLC

In loving memory of my parents, Muriel Zimmerman and Harry Slochower, my beloved maternal grandmother, Belle Zimmerman, and my children, Jesse, Alison, and Avi. My delicious grandchildren, Harry, Adi, Shai, Eitan, Iris, Elisha, and very little Rosie have given me such extraordinary joy.

# Contents

*List of contributors*                                                    *xi*
*Preface: Nancy McWilliams*                                               *xiii*
*Acknowledgments*                                                         *xvi*
*Introduction*                                                           *xvii*

**PART 1   BEYOND BINARIES: HOLDING IN A
            RELATIONAL CONTEXT**                                           **1**

Introduction: Dodi Goldman                                                 3

1   Bridging the gap: Developing a relational holding model                7

2   Revisiting the maternal metaphor: A long view                         20

3   Resist this                                                           30

4   Going too far: Relational heroines and relational excess              40

5   A few regrets                                                         52


**PART 2   PUSHING THE ENVELOPE: HOW FAR IS TOO FAR?**                     **65**

Introduction: Andrea Celenza                                              67

6   The analyst's secret delinquencies                                    71

7   Ghosts that haunt                                                     85

8   Sequels                                                               99

**PART 3  BEYOND THE CONSULTING ROOM: MOURNING,
ACTUALITY, AND ILLUSIONS                                  121**

Introduction: Irwin Kula                                      123

9  Getting better all the time?                               129

10  Out of the analytic shadow                                143

11  The absent witness: Mourning, virtually                   161

12  Factions are back                                         169

13  Creating inner space: The psychoanalytic writer          188


*Afterword*                                                   *201*
*References*                                                  *204*
*Index*                                                       *222*

# Contributors

Nancy McWilliams is Visiting Professor Emerita at Rutgers Graduate School of Applied & Professional Psychology and has a private practice in Lambertville, NJ. She is author of four textbooks (on psychoanalytic diagnosis, case formulation, therapy, and supervision) and is co-editor of both editions of the *Psychodynamic Diagnostic Manual*. A former president of the Society for Psychoanalysis and Psychoanalytic Psychotherapy of the American Psychological Association, she is a member of the Austen Riggs Center Board of Trustees. Her books are available in 20 languages, and she has taught in 30 countries.

Dodi Goldman, Ph.D. is a Training and Supervising Analyst and Faculty at the William Alanson White Institute. He authored, *In Search of the Real: The Origins and Originality of D.W. Winnicott,* edited and wrote an introduction to *In One's Bones: The Clinical Genius of D.W. Winnicott,* and is the former book review editor of the journal *Contemporary Psychoanalysis*. His book, *A Beholder's Share: Essays on Winnicott and the Psychoanalytic Imagination*, won the 2017 Gradiva Award for Best Psychoanalytic Book. A forthcoming book, *A Shimmering Landscape: The Imaginative and Actual in Psychic Life* will be published by Routledge in 2025. Dodi maintains a private practice and study groups in Manhattan and Great Neck, NY.

Andrea Celenza, Ph.D. is a Training and Supervising Analyst at the Boston Psychoanalytic Society and Institute and Assistant Clinical Professor at Harvard Medical School. She is also Adjunct Faculty at the NYU Post-Doctoral Program in Psychoanalysis and The Florida Psychoanalytic Center. She has written numerous papers on love, sexuality, and psychoanalysis and is on the Editorial Board of JAPA. She has two online courses and is the recipient of several awards. Her writings have been translated into Italian, Spanish, Korean, Russian, and Farsi. Her third book, entitled, *Transference, Love, and Being: Essential Essays from the Field,* was published in 2022 by Routledge and she has two forthcoming works, *Erotic Transferences: A Contemporary Introduction* (Routledge, July 2024) and a co-edited volume (with Murray Schwartz) of American Imago on Perverse Scenarios. Dr. Celenza is in private practice in Lexington, Massachusetts, USA.

Irwin Kula is a seventh generation rabbi, President Emeritus of Clal— The National Jewish Center for Learning and Leadership and author of the award-winning book *Yearnings: Embracing the Sacred Messiness of Life.* He works with organizations, foundations, and businesses around the world at the intersection of religion, innovation, and the sciences of human flourishing. A commentator in both new and traditional media, he is co-founder with Craig Hatkoff and the late Professor Clay Christensen of the Disruptor Foundation whose mission is to advance disruptive innovation theory and its application in societal critical domains. Irwin lives in NYC. His most important teachers and greatest joys are his wife of 41 years, his two daughters and sons-in-law, and his two grandchildren, the elder of whom regularly says, "I can do it by my own self."

# Preface

*Nancy McWilliams, Ph.D., ABPP*

Joyce Slochower has devoted much of her career to writing about what is both obvious and invisible. In this compilation of articles authored over several decades, some substantially rethought and revised, she wrestles with one after another aspect of psychoanalytic practice that has been implicit, unelaborated, obfuscated, or veiled by taboo—those phenomenon that break into the sacred spaces in which psychoanalytic consultations take place. Her explorations involve areas that all therapists struggle with as we confront the myriad ways that people suffer psychologically, and as we try to evaluate the multitude of contradictory prescriptions we receive from mentors and colleagues about how best to help our patients.

This book is particularly engaging because it allows readers to witness the evolution of the thinking of an influential relational analyst. I read many of these articles when they were first published, but they are especially compelling when framed, as they are here, by the author's personal reflections on the emergence of her ideas and by the trenchant observations of the scholars who introduce each section. Hindsight, as we often quip, can be much more acute than foresight; retrospective compilations like this allow readers to comprehend not only particular concepts relevant to their work but also why those concepts emerged when and where they did.

Although we were trained in different institutes and influenced by mentors with different views, I have long felt an affinity for Joyce's work and have come to know her well over the last couple of decades. Her story resembles that of one of my psychoanalytic heroes, Frieda Fromm-Reichmann (see Hornstein, 2000). Like Fromm-Reichmann, Joyce was raised in a warm Jewish family that prized intellectual curiosity, education, compassion, social service, and moral commitment. She grew up struggling with the great human questions and watching her parents do the same. She evolved into a moralist who is not moralistic, an authority who is not authoritarian, an expert who views expertise with suspicion.

Joyce is more interested in what behavior helps one's client than in what practices comport with prevailing orthodoxies—including relational orthodoxies. She has never identified uncritically with any theorist—not even with her beloved Winnicott, whom she admires but also takes to task in several areas. Despite being central to the inception and development of the relational movement in psychoanalysis, she has not been self-promotional in the sense of seeking the status of a charismatic leader in that community. She has never presented her own ideas as unprecedented or transformational. She prefers unpretentious roles such as raiser of questions and complicator of assumptions, and she can frequently be found doing the grunt work necessary for accomplishing goals that are important to the professional communities that matter to her.

For many years, I have been interested in the differences between wisdom and knowledge. Although this book is full of both, its primary contribution is its wisdom, the capacity that Sternberg (2003, p. xviii) defined as "the value-laden application of tacit knowledge not only for one's own benefit . . . but also for the benefit of others, in order to attain a common good." Cynthia Baum-Baicker's interviews of analysts whose communities regard them as "wise elders" (Baum-Baicker & Sisti, 2012) uncovered themes in their lives and careers of openness to experience, capacity to tolerate uncertainty and paradox, sensitivity to complexity, respect for conventional rules coexisting with the willingness to challenge them, and a sense of balance between immersion in experience and critical reflection.

These characteristics of psychoanalytic wise elders are visible throughout Joyce's work, even the work of her younger professional self. They describe her engagement with all the areas she explores in this collection of her contributions, whether she is addressing how to integrate Winnicott's conception of holding within a relational sensibility, or exposing analysts' private lapses from full attention to the patient, or exploring the limits and biases in her individual vision and the perspective of relational psychoanalysis generally, or speculating about the psychological impacts of the recent pandemic, or elucidating the process of writing itself.

The virtue of humility emerges repeatedly in scholarly writings about the nature of wisdom, an observation that prompts me to remind readers that it was the relational movement that put the attitude of "not knowing" at the forefront of psychoanalytic practice. Among those who pioneered relational psychoanalysis, Slochower has been particularly suspicious of analytic generalizations about what is always the "right" thing to do. She takes human fallibility for granted and would be uncomfortable if anyone used her own contributions to develop a new orthodoxy. Although her personal style is hardly self-abnegating, she holds rigorously to an ideal of modesty about knowledge claims and is allergic to intellectual arrogance.

Consistent with Erikson's (1950) ideas about generativity in one's older years, Joyce is at a time in her life when mature scholars become particularly invested in passing on what they have learned to clinicians who are newer to our strange profession. For decades now, she has been teaching, supervising, and mentoring, always with a view toward fostering each student's authentic competence rather than promoting compliant acceptance of her own ideas. This book can be seen as a kind of love letter to the next generation of analysts. I encourage you to read it as such, to enjoy its witty and accessible conversational style, and to benefit from its wisdom.

# Acknowledgments

Even if one has a room of one's own within which to write, multiple influences—sometimes ghosts—hopefully benign ones—accompany that process. Mine are multiple.

I begin with my psychoanalyst parents, Muriel Zimmerman and Harry Slochower, along with my maternal grandmother, Belle Zimmerman; no, they didn't always provide the holding I needed. But they gave me a lot and modeled an ethical way of being in the world. Their influence, however, was indirect. It was my patients who really taught me how to do this work, how to think and rethink therapeutic process and consider my own contribution to moments of impasse.

I've been blessed with many wonderful supervisees, students, study, and supervision group members whose questions and wisdom have pushed me beyond my own psychoanalytic framework. Especially valuable were the creative and critical thoughts of close friends and colleagues who generously read and responded to portions of these essays. In alphabetical order, they are Lew Aron, Marty Frommer, Sue Grand, Ruth Gruenthal, Margerie Kalb, and Ruth Stein (now gone but a forever influence). Each brought their creativity and deep thinking to this material in ways that enriched and complicated it. I thank my musicologist son, Jesse Rodin, for his sharp literary eye (and his gift for creative titles). I'm also grateful to my editor, Don Stern, for his support and interest in this project.

# Introduction

My entry into the field of psychoanalysis was, to understate, overdetermined: Both of my parents (and my stepfather) were analysts. Psychoanalysis was childhood's backdrop; clinical jargon punctuated dinner table conversations. Since my parents' offices were in our apartment, I was an occasional witness to psychoanalytic ritual. Patients sometimes passed me in the hall on their way into sessions, only to disappear behind thick, soundproof doors. What *were* they talking about? I have but the fuzziest of memories, but I'm sure I had plenty of fantasies about the mysterious goings-on as unintelligible voices rose and fell.

In addition, my parents didn't always heed Winnicott's (1963a) warning that "Parents who interpret the unconscious to their children are in for a bad time" (p. 251). I didn't appreciate their interpretations, but I did wonder whether they were right. Rather than turning me against the field or against my parents, their interpretations left me intrigued. Psychoanalysis was thus both tantalizing and off-limits; perhaps I could get—and give—what I imagined their patients got by way of understanding and help.

And there was more. My father, an academic-turned-analyst, had been deeply involved in the (socialist/communist) anti-Hitler movement in the 1930s. His fierce hatred of fascism made him a victim of McCarthy's Red Scare attack on academics: He was fired by Brooklyn College for refusing to names. My dad's refusal to inform inspired me; here was a position of integrity worth emulating. My mother, while more politically cautious, was equally fierce in her commitment to personal and professional ethics. Her insistence on "doing the right thing" was similarly inspiring (see the Afterword).

I entered analytic training firmly identified with my parents' Freudian orientation. The certainty it offered was comforting; there were rules to follow, a right way and a wrong way to do things. But certainty came at a price; over time, its constricting effect began to outweigh its value. I didn't want to answer *every* question with a question. I wanted to be freer to "be" within the therapeutic setting and to name what I saw. I chafed at my Freudian supervisor's insistence that I maintain rigid boundaries even when my patient seemed to need something very different.

Looking for a therapeutic alternative, I sought out an interpersonal supervisor. But staying in the moment was differently limiting; it skipped over my patient's early history. Pregnant with my first child, I received Winnicott's (1964) *The Child, the Family, and the Outside World* from a family friend (ironically, a classical Freudian analyst—Ruth Lax). This was a prescient gift; Winnicott's work offered a compelling alternative to the classical model. I read every Winnicott piece I could get my hands on.

At once quirky and maternal, Winnicott evoked a vision of affective responsivity, of a new, improved mother/father. That vision generated a powerful response. If the analyst symbolically can become the mother, the possibility of reworking early trauma increases enormously: What cannot be remembered can be reexperienced and then repaired; the patient can be a baby again, but with a better, more responsive (symbolic) mother.

Winnicott's ideas about transitionality, illusion, paradox, hate, and the move from object relating to object usage, in tandem with his vision of regression to dependence and therapeutic repair, accompanied me as I encountered the relational perspective. Trying to bridge the apparently incompatible, I developed what I called a relational holding model and applied it to a range of clinical issues. *Holding and Psychoanalysis* (1996c, 2014d) contains much of that work.

*Psychoanalysis and the Unspoken* is a compilation—and in many instances a significant reworking—of essays written over a more than 30-year period. It addresses many issues beyond holding, all organized around the theme of psychoanalytic ideals and their limits. In it, I aim to identify and query our field's clinical and theoretical underbellies and open a reflective space within which to name and explore unspoken or underspoken aspects of our thinking and personhood as they shape, develop, and limit our clinical work.

I've been blessed with many wonderful colleagues and friends, four of whom have generously contributed to this volume. *Psychoanalysis and the Unspoken*'s Preface is written by my esteemed colleague Nancy McWilliams. Nancy's wise, sophisticated perspective locates the book's themes within a broader theoretical/clinical envelope. Dodi Goldman, an important Winnicott scholar, introduces Part 1. Andrea Celenza, an expert in boundary violations, introduces Part 2, in which I address the violations that permeate the field. Irwin Kula, a rabbi with an extraordinarily literate psychoanalytic sensibility, frames Part 3, where I explore other collisions between the psychoanalytic ideal and actuality (see also *Psychoanalytic Collisions*, 2006b, 2014b; 2015b).

## Overview

**Part 1, Beyond Binaries: Holding in a Relational Context** reflects on my (now almost "40-year") immersion, first in Winnicottian and then in relational thinking. **Chapter 1** (*Bridging the gap: Developing a relational holding model*) describes my early understanding of relational holding and its clinical function; **Chapter 2** (*Revisiting the maternal metaphor: A long view*) revisits that model from a contemporary perspective and argues for the inclusion of an updated baby metaphor in contemporary thinking. **Chapter 3** (*Resist this*) reconsiders the concept of resistance and argues for its inclusion within a relational framework. **Chapter 4** (*Going too far: Relational heroines and relational excess*) critiques the concept of analytic mutuality and the idealization of self-disclosure and enactment. **Chapter 5** (*A few regrets*) turns that critique on my own theory of relational holding and identifies what it misses or minimizes.

**Part 2, Pushing the Envelope: How Far Is Too Far?** turns a lens on our profession's underbelly. **Chapter 6** (*The analyst's secret delinquencies*) explores the dynamics driving professional "delinquencies"—ways in which we privilege our own needs and "steal" time or attention from our patient. **Chapter 7** (*Ghosts that haunt*) addresses what is, perhaps, the field's most problematic and disturbing issue—the prevalence of sexual boundary violations. I focus *not* on the dynamics of the violating analyst but on how we who are indirect witnesses assimilate these breaches. **Chapter 8** (*Sequels*) explores another edge of our professional boundaries—nonsexual post-treatment friendships between ex-analysands and their former analysts. Here, I revisit the termination ideal and go out on a bit of a limb by proposing that post-treatment friendships can embody a positive element.

**Part 3, Beyond the Consulting Room: Mourning, Actuality, and Illusions** is written from my current perspective as an older analyst with nearly 40 years of clinical experience behind me and, inevitably, less than that ahead. **Chapter 9** (*Getting better all the time?*) addresses the analyst's experience of aging and its collision with our fantasy of perpetually going on being. **Chapter 10** (*Out of the analytic shadow*) focuses on the holding function of mourning and memorial ritual across the lifespan. **Chapter 11** (*The absent witness: Mourning, virtually*) brings things into the current moment by exploring the impact of Covid and virtual treatment on clinical process and, particularly, on mourning. **Chapter 12** (*Factions are back*) steps back from the personal and describes the intertheoretical tribalism that has dominated our field since its beginnings. Can we move beyond these splits and toward an overarching professional identity? **Chapter 13** (*Creating inner space: The psychoanalytic writer*) looks at how creative illusions allow us to enter the writing process.

The **Afterword** (*Against the grain: On challenging assumptions, bridging theories, practicing self-critique, exposing underbellies, and doing the right thing*) briefly reflects on the personal origins of these themes.

# Part 1

# Beyond Binaries

## Holding in a Relational Context

# Introduction

## Dodi Goldman

D. W. Winnicott once famously warned his students: "What you get out of me you will have to pick out of chaos" (Grolnick & Barkin, 1978, p.37). And because he offered us, his students, such an array of potentially generative metaphors, pick we do. For Joyce Slochower, it is Winnicott's notion of maternal holding that captivates her clinical imagination and upon which she builds a creative synthesis all her own.

It is fitting Slochower brings together her writings on "holding" under the general banner of "beyond binaries." One reason Winnicott remained a somewhat quixotic figure for so long was precisely because his vision cut across the polarizing dichotomies of his day: People are both innovative symbol makers and biologically driven organisms, accounts of human behavior include both maturational processes and facilitating environments, the self is a content of a purported mental apparatus but also an overarching locus of experience. For Winnicott, even what we call "environment," is never simply and solely "outside" the individual. To a certain extent, we create our own personal environment even as there is an actual external provision, which may or may not be good enough or made good-enough imaginative use of. What makes Winnicott both maddeningly elusive and excitingly generative is that such paradoxes are the animating spirit behind his sensibility.

Some of the dichotomies Winnicott approached paradoxically, Slochower engages dialectically. She believes clinical theories are, in her words, "almost always formulated in opposition to clashing ones, an ongoing series of correctives that frequently become pendulum swings."

What sets these pendulum swings in motion is a tendency—*across all our theories*—toward excess. Slochower observes how substantive critiques by American relationalists generated valuable correctives to facets

DOI: 10.4324/9781032691534-2

of classical thinking. But like every theory, the new vision itself became vulnerable to caricature.

Slochower notes, for example, that relational analysts virtually discarded the classical notion of "resistance." Might this be, she wonders, a new form of resistance among her own colleagues? Whereas earlier, analysts had been unwilling to locate resistance anywhere *but* inside the patient, relational analysts viewed resistance to be inherently dyadic rather than individually derived. And so, Slochower invites "the idea of the difficult patient— separate from the difficult dyad—back into relational space."

As Slochower set out to reassess such foreclosures of relational thinking, she found in Winnicott's "holding" a metaphor well suited to describe what she feared was getting lost. Winnicott rarely expressed the powerful metaphors he fashioned as exact logical concepts. They were, as Harry Guntrip (1975) noted early on, "imaginative hypotheses that challenged one to explore further" (p.155). Slochower makes her own imaginative use of "holding," no longer associating it solely to situations of regression to dependence. Instead, she forthrightly challenges prevailing assumptions, including her own, to question what works, and what potentially impedes, analytic engagement.

"Holding," for Slochower, serves not only as a way of describing a particular phase in a child's emergence from an undifferentiated state during which the foundation of a primal sense of well-being is laid down—in Winnicott's words, "a blueprint for existentialism." It becomes a broader and powerful symbol of all that is potentially eclipsed by the relational turn: Attention to interiority, the developmental roots and fragility of inner solidity, the healthy need for privacy and aloneness, sensitivity to shaming. Seemingly "correct" interpretations, Slochower recognizes, are often not very well-disguised accusations. Furthermore, an analyst's excessive expressivity can do damage when it fails to adequately resonate with the patient's own experience.

I read Slochower's work as an act of rebalancing. It is also somewhat of a balancing act as she strives to reconcile an American relationalist emphasis on mutual engagement with Winnicott's attunement to what is developmentally necessary to make such engagement possible. Slochower presents us with a version of "holding" not only from the point of view of a "knowing" analyst but as a vital shared illusion generated between patient and analyst. Even as she forthrightly reassesses what is potentially foreclosed by the movement of which she is very much a part, Slochower also candidly recalibrates herself.

A supervisee of Winnicott's once attended a talk he gave about "knowledge." She was quite familiar with Winnicott's non-linear way of speaking but felt that on this particular occasion he was going on in a "particularly tortuous, roundabout fashion." Perhaps it was an urge to help him out that prompted her to rise from the audience and summarize what she "knew" he was trying to say by asking something along the lines of: "If, to have genuine personal significance, people must discover things for themselves, how can an analyst ever directly interpret anything? Is making a premature interpretation a spoiling kind of activity?" Without hesitating, Winnicott replied: "Your question is a better answer than any I could give."

What was striking was what happened next. It was as if the very matter under discussion—"knowledge"—was enacted within the audience. As soon as the supervisee sat down, a hum of "What did she say?" broke out. It seemed to her that many in the audience had not really been listening as they were too preoccupied with their own thoughts. Suddenly, someone else in the audience took it upon himself to repeat and "explain" what she had just said. Irritated he was misrepresenting her; she felt an urge to correct him. But then, she recalls, she "caught sight of Winnicott looking at me, frowning slightly, raising a finger to his lips, narrowing his eyes . . ." In a flash, she understood his communication to her: What anyone understands at any particular moment is the best that person can muster given their circumstances and personal history. She realized her task at the moment was to bear—Slochower might say, "bracket"—being misunderstood (Issroff, 2005, pp.21–22).

The Winnicott that emerges from this vignette, however, is only one version of Winnicott. Anyone who has read his personal correspondences or the reviews he wrote for medical journals knows full well how direct and frontal he could be in leveling criticism and his prickliness when his contributions were overlooked by colleagues. Winnicott, like Slochower, reminds us that there is a time and a place for everything.

Some analysts find Winnicott difficult to digest, while others find his sensibility naturally appealing. But "appeal" or even "influence," doesn't occur only from the "outside-in." It reveals an inner readiness to take in and elaborate offerings that then enrich inner experience. As the Gospels say, the Word can fall on stony ground, or it might find rich soil and bear fruit.

Original ideas require a receptive ear. But receptivity implies a person pre-reflexively inclined toward the idea. We "hear and apprehend only what we already half-know," Thoreau wrote in his journals (Shepard, 1961, p.212).

In the following chapters, Slochower offers us a glimpse into how her own receptive ear and inner readiness aligned her with Winnicott's sensibility. And since Winnicott preferred to be used rather than be right, I can't help but imagine he'd take pleasure encountering Slochower using him while being very much herself.

# Chapter 1

# Bridging the gap
## Developing a relational holding model

Winnicott "is" my psychoanalytic hero. Evocative and inspiring, his vision of maternal (analytic) repair suggested that the patient could be a baby again, but with a better, more responsive mother. That vision invited a significant reformulation of therapeutic process and had a powerful effect on psychoanalytic thinking.

Lodging the analyst's therapeutic stance in diagnosis, Winnicott distinguished the needs of neurotic patients (who could be treated classically) and depressive patients (for whom the object's survival is central) from those of schizoid and psychotic patients. Today we would probably call the latter group borderline. This group cannot assimilate "ordinary" analytic work—especially interpretations—because the false (caretaker) self dominates; in the absence of access to true self experience, no real change accrues. These patients need to access and relive early trauma in the presence of a holding analyst who permits a regression to dependence by establishing a space protected from environmental impingements (Winnicott, 1960a, 1963a). When early trauma enters a benign analytic relationship, developmental processes can restart and revitalize the true self.

During a regression to dependence, emotional and sometimes literal support might be required; interpretations are used (if at all) to support the analytic holding function rather than to stimulate insight or break through resistance.

Winnicott envisioned this therapeutic process, then, as symbolic maternal repair for what we'd now call relational trauma. His developmental metaphor changed the clinical landscape by focusing not on the repeated relationship but on the needed one (S. Stern, 1994). He named something that had remained largely unspoken: the clinical value of empathic responsivity.

DOI: 10.4324/9781032691534-3

Now it was theorized: Dependence wasn't defensive because early need was real and needed real repair.

There was far more to the Winnicottian vision than regression to dependence (see Goldman, 2017, for a wonderfully perceptive review of his work). For Winnicott, regression to dependence was not itself a clinical endpoint but instead an essential step en route to contacting the true self and working through anger at the original parental failure. Its aim was the establishment of a two-person relationship. Here, though, I focus on Winnicott's understanding of the therapeutic holding function.

Winnicott viewed holding as less a technical prescription than a metaphor for the "early environment" dimension of analytic work. The ordinary devoted mother held the baby over time by providing in a highly sensitive way what was needed. Just what this looked like, of course, depended on the patient; Winnicott anticipated the intersubjective turn when he (1970) wrote, "if a mother has eight children, there are eight mothers" (p. 40).

Perhaps our most evocative description of Winnicott's way of holding comes from his analyst patient Margaret Little:

> . . . metaphorically he was holding the situation, giving support, keeping contact on every level with whatever was going on in and around the patient, and in relationship to him . . . Literally through for many hours he held my hands, clasped between his, almost like an umbilical cord, while I lay, often hidden beneath the blanket, silent, withdrawn, inert, in panic, rage, or tears, asleep, sometimes dreaming.
>
> (Little, 1990, p. 44)

This idealized vision of analytic process (and babyhood) is alive and well today. The morning of this writing, a businesswoman patient who usually experiences herself as enormously grown-up and feels me to be a helpful consultant-peer sat down and said, "I have to tell you that I feel like curling up into a ball and weeping like a little girl. I've been waiting so long to get here. I can't believe it's only been a week and I can't believe how dependent I feel." She didn't stay there, but for some moments she touched a baby wish, and as it came affectively alive I resonated both with her wish and with the possibility of meeting it. This phenomenon is so common as to be commonplace, though its place in our theorizing varies widely.

## Winnicott and the relational critique

Winnicott's romantic analytic vision wasn't universally embraced. It seemed to conflate wish and need, as if repair could replace the analysis of conflict. From a classical perspective, it omitted the dynamics of aggression and envy—of attachment to bad objects. For interpersonal and social constructivist writers, the maternal metaphor (patient/baby and analyst/mother) itself was problematic (e.g., Aron, 1992; Hoffman, 1991; Mitchell, 1984, 1988, 1993; D. B. Stern, 1992). The assumptions on which it lay—analytic certainty, knowledge, power, and the possibility of delineating historical "truth"—were sharply challenged. Elaborating the social constructivist critique, relationalists reconceived analytic history as a shared narrative developed between analyst and patient. The relational analyst is embroiled in, rather than residing above, therapeutic process. She's neither omniscient nor omnipotent; her personhood inevitably disrupts the maternal illusion. Further, the idea that she can repair the patient's past embodies far too much certainty, both about what happened and about the analyst's capacity to "correct" that past.

From this perspective, holding obfuscates the actual. Clinical action lies instead in the analysis of (re)enactments; both (adult) parties become caught up in replaying and then unpacking early relational dynamics. In this mutual, if asymmetrical, relationship, the patient can—at least at moments—recognize the analyst's subjectivity. The relational patient, then, is anything but a baby. What *was* no longer *is*; she brings her adult self, with all its attendant conflicts and complex ways of experiencing things, to the consulting room. When enacted, developmental illusions create an "as if" therapeutic situation that locks the patient into a position of helpless dependence while encouraging the analyst's grandiosity.

Adding to the relational critique of Winnicott were voices rooted in feminist thinking (e.g., Bassin, Honey & Kaplan, 1994; Benjamin, 1986; Chodorow & Contratto, 1982; Harris, 1997). Challenging the idealization of motherhood and its associated demand for maternal self-abnegation, they noted that traditional views of motherhood exculpate the father and "deposit" all the child's pathology in the maternal lap. This position forecloses the idea, no matter the experience, of mother-as-person. Feminist psychoanalysts pushed back against this maternal ideal and sounded a clarion call for the explicit recognition of the mother/analyst's subjectivity (see Benjamin,

1988). Visions of analyst-as-earthmother negate that subjectivity, along with the patient/baby's capacity to see and know. And they ignore the preoedipal father.

Winnicott (1971) believed that the child gradually becomes capable of experiencing the mother as *other*—that is, as an external (rather than a subjective) object—because she survives the child's (fantasied) destruction of her. Benjamin uses this idea but pushes beyond the Winnicottian perspective by showing that the mother's subjectivity was essential to the child's developing the capacity for intersubjective relatedness, that is, for mutual recognition (see McKay, 2019).

Despite his idealized vision of the holding analyst, Winnicott (1947) was also aware of the strain inherent in analytic (and maternal) holding. But he believed that the analyst—and mother—could bear that strain without expressing it.

I wasn't so sure. As a young mother struggling to balance career and parenthood, the feminist critique hit home. I wanted, and felt I had to, do it all—and do it awfully well. Then I discovered a children's album recorded by American singer Marlo Thomas. It was titled *Free to Be . . . You and Me* and included a song whose chorus was "Mommies are people, people with children." The sense, finally, of recognition. (I still know all the words.) Today, I think it's shocking how shocking those words were. Yet now, more than three decades later, I occasionally fight the impulse to sing it to my adult, married children. For while mommies eventually become subjects to their children, it's the rare child who steadily sustains that awareness. And in many ways, the same is true of patients vis-à-vis their analysts.

## A relational holding model

Aiming to bridge the Winnicottian and relational perspectives, I spent several decades developing what I came to call a relational holding model (Slochower, 1991, 1992, 1993, 1994, 1996 a, b, c, 2006c, 2014b, 2018a). Steve Mitchell invited me to put that work in the Relational Perspectives Book Series; *Holding and Psychoanalysis: A Relational Perspective* thus came to be under his extraordinary editorship.

My premise was this: While intersubjective exchange is a relational goal, it's not always a therapeutic reality. In the absence of a capacity to tolerate explicit I-Thou engagement, holding becomes essential. Analytic holding blurs the permeable boundary between patient and analyst and buffers the impact of the analyst's otherness while creating a wider space that can expand a patient's access to her interiority. Within that wider space, an illusion of analytic attunement—variously shaped—remains unchallenged.

Holding, then, represents the analyst's attempt—never completely successful—to remain within a patient's subjective frame. I recognize, name, and accept my patient's feelings, whatever their shape, without countering or interpreting what I hear. And, most importantly, I neither collapse nor retaliate. Holding thus embodies a double communication: I'm affected by, but not engulfed, obliterated, or enraged, by you.

The holding metaphor, then, embodies resonant connection. It's embedded in a benign, generative idealization that repairs without the kickback of devaluation. Like Sandler's (1960) background of safety, holding represents an underlying element that's also present as a silent background during explicitly interactive clinical work.

I view holding not as a one-person clinical process but as one emerging within an overarching intersubjective frame. Analytic holding is itself an enactment: Rather than "deciding" or "choosing" to hold based on a clinical (diagnostic) assessment, the move toward holding emerges out of a kind of nonverbal dance. My patient signals her intolerance of my separateness via explicit and nonverbal reactions to my input; I (sometimes consciously, sometimes procedurally) respond to that intolerance by moving toward a more containing position.

But it's not only I who hold; my patient picks up on what we—or she—can't tolerate and brackets it. A mutually protective space emerges, one characterized *not* by dissociation but by a need/desire to keep the process going. Mutual bracketing buffers what could otherwise be derailing, and the work deepens.

At moments, holding helps my patient down-regulate. Down-regulation may involve Bion's (1962) container function; flooding hatred becomes irritation; overwhelming longing becomes wished-for connection. Alternatively, down-regulation sometimes occurs via the interactive dyadic dance Beebe and Lachmann (1994) discuss. Together, patient and analyst quiet the intense emotion evoked; distress gradually diminishes, and things settle a bit.

But holding isn't enough. Whether we identify the holding dimension as figure or as ground, we (I) do far more than hold, and the rest of what we do counts a lot; interpretation, confrontation, and play are all central dimensions of analytic work. Here, though, I underscore the need for moments of resonant recognition, not only in analysis, but across the lifetime (see Chapter 10). This is where the shadow holding element comes in: It guides us on a procedural level with regard to when and how we enter the clinical dialogue, how directly and how deeply.

## Holding and analytic bracketing

Analytic holding is always partial; even when we hold, aspects of our subjectivity leak into the treatment space. But while we can't delete ourselves, we *can* work to contain what's disruptive while bracketing, i.e., by neither expressing nor deleting our disjunctive subjectivity. The latter is crucial; if we negate our experience (deny/disavow that we're feeling what we're feeling), clinical process is likely to freeze and result in a problematic rather than workable enactment.

Bracketing, then, alludes to the doubleness of the holding experience, the there-but-not-there quality of my subjectivity. I may well feel stressed, tired, impatient—even angry—in ways that would be disturbing, anxiety arousing, or otherwise upsetting to my patient. Bracketing means privately noting but then trying to set aside my reaction. It does *not* mean disavowing or denying it.

It's difficult to describe all this without making it sound deliberate, even choreographed. But shifts in and out of a holding metaphor are anything but. On one level, I move toward holding based on my clinical/theoretical point of entrée. On another, this shift is procedural, a spontaneous reaction to that which I've not yet identified. On yet another, holding reflects a mutual, dissociated dyadic dance. And to complicate things even further, some of the time I—we all—fail when we try to hold, because we think we know what's needed but don't; because we're in the throes of an enactment, selfobject failure, or other kind of misattunement. Or because there's simply too much for us to hold (Slochower, 1996c, 2014c). Further, we can't bracket what we don't know we're feeling (and we can't hold what we don't know needs holding). Additionally, many patients are pretty perceptive (sometimes more than we'd like) and pick up aspects of our subjectivity despite our attempts to bracket.

### Who's doing the bracketing?

Both of us: When my patient needs *not* to know something about me, she does as much, even more, bracketing than I do. She shields herself (unconsciously or procedurally) from those aspects of my otherness (my variability, reactivity, and so on) that would disrupt the sense of resonance on which she relies.

So, *bracketing takes two*. The idea of mutual bracketing moves holding out of the analyst's corner and into dyadic space. It reverses the asymmetry originally associated with the Winnicottian metaphor and relocates holding into the relational arena.

Here's an example: I was a young analyst, eight months pregnant with my third child. Feeling I could no longer wait for my patient Jonathan, neither very ill nor especially dissociative, to address the obvious, I said, "There's something we need to talk about." Fully expecting him to acknowledge that he hadn't wanted to bring up my pregnancy but of course had noticed, I was surprised to see him do a double take and virtually fall back in his chair, stunned.

Jonathan's need to see us as a couple had foreclosed his conscious awareness of my pregnancy, a most concrete indication of my otherness. He also excluded what it represented (the prospect of a symbolic sibling, not to mention my shadow husband—the unseen sexual partner who fathered this child). He thereby sustained an essential experience of togetherness with me. Ours wasn't a holding space reminiscent of the nursery, though. Jonathan felt me to be a peer/older sister who was identified with his needs. An element of twinship merged with maternal longings to render me "a woman, but just like him." Hence, not pregnant. And as much as I consciously wanted to be seen in my expectant state, perhaps on another level I unconsciously supported his bracketing via my wish to protect our relationship (and my baby) by leaving the latter outside therapeutic space.

Eventually Jonathan and I talked about what he had needed to miss and why. Our conversations filled in and thickened the therapeutic dialogue, but I'm pretty sure they couldn't have taken place had I insistently introduced my pregnancy early on.

### What holding looks like

I don't assume that holding is what's needed in each treatment. I turn to holding only when my patient is consistently unable to accept and work with *or* reject my perspective while sustaining her own. I'm not referring to whether my patient accepts what I say: A loud "No damn way, you're

wrong" may signal a new kind of mutual engagement that will open analytic process.

But when my patient consistently reacts to my "separate" input by shut-
ting down, I sit up, therapeutically speaking. I ask myself whether I'm off
base, whether we're involved in a potentially useful—or problematic—
reenactment. Is my patient reacting to my being too much like "old objects"
or too different from them?

A background awareness of her reaction to evidence of my "otherness"—
my "separate" thoughts, reactions, and feelings—informs these shifts. It's
only when I can't usefully unpack an enactment that I move toward holding
and try to help her feel seen, not from the outside in, but from the inside
out (Bromberg, 1991). Resonating with her feeling or perception, containing the "but" that would be implicit in my attempt to interpret or deepen
her understanding ("but you could experience or see it differently"), I try
to give her more room within which to identify or amplify a nascent or
partially articulated experience (Slochower, 2004).

Am I off base, emotionally or dynamically? Are we involved in a potentially useful or very problematic reenactment? Is my patient reacting to my
being too much like "old objects" or too different from them? I hold by trying to name her experience without countering, complicating, or interpreting the dynamics associated with it. Privileging access to private space and
allowing my patient to feel out the edges of her own insideness helps her
more easily access interior process.

Winnicott (1958) reminded us that the capacity to be alone is first established when the baby can be comfortably alone in Mother's presence. Many
adult experiences, including creative activity and non-anxious aloneness,
are based on a capacity to sustain one's sense of interiority. Interiority
(Slochower, 1999) alludes to a sense of personal solidity within which
subjective experience and privacy are taken for granted. A solid sense of
interiority is a prerequisite for mutual engagement; without it, the other's
perspective is derailing.

While holding is traditionally associated with regression to dependence
(i.e., with an intense reliance on the analyst), the holding thread can be
found in clinical situations characterized *not* by early need but by difficulties sustaining a solid sense of one's own experience. I illustrate a different
kind of clinical moment characterized by holding.

Samuel's well-meaning professional parents tended to blur the line
between their clinical and parental roles. They were hyper-attuned to his

feelings, often telling Samuel what he felt before he himself knew. Samuel tended to adopt their assessment of him as his own (see Kohut, 1977, pp. 146–151, on the children of psychoanalysts).

Chronically confused about what was "his," Samuel typically began sessions with a tentative, vague description of his day and feelings. But he soon trailed off, unable to further name his experience. I tried to help; I asked, for example, what the upset feeling was like, where he located it in his body, when else he had felt it. Samuel seemed puzzled by my questions, unable to elaborate more than he already had. He was equally uncertain about what might have set off his reaction, offering many possibilities with no sense of conviction about what felt right. When I tentatively sketched out my understanding of his experience, Samuel quickly settled upon it as *the* answer in a way that felt more compliant than authentic. If I pointed to his need to please others (including me) at the expense of his own subjectivity, Samuel would agree but then wait for me to provide a solution. Thus, even as I laid out the dilemma before us, I reenacted Samuel's parents' knowing position, leaving him the helpless child, dependent on my analytic acumen and still confused about himself.

Now aware of this, I shifted away from active engagement. This shift had both deliberate and procedural elements. In part, I told myself to wait and sat on my impulse to actively offer my own thoughts; but on another level, I found myself *feeling* reflective and receptive rather than eager to engage in active dialogue. I began asking Samuel what he made of his feelings and didn't fill in the silences that followed. Samuel initially reacted with anxiety to my questions, unable to shift into himself. I acknowledged his discomfort but refrained from naming his experience in ways that went beyond his own descriptions. Very gradually, Samuel began to lapse into silence in sessions. Initially, I found these silences difficult to tolerate; I worried that Samuel was complying with my idea about what he needed rather than exploring his own subjectivity. Occasionally, I responded to my discomfort by giving voice to my ideas about Samuel's process. But my feeling of therapeutic efficacy gave way to an uncomfortable awareness that Samuel was again establishing me as the arbiter of his internal state, agreeing with my understanding in a reflexive rather than integrated way.

Over months, Samuel's comfort with silence increased. This was mainly evident in a shift in his posture on the couch. He had previously lain somewhat stiffly and self-consciously, his head tilted slightly to the side and toward me, as if awaiting my input. Now he began settling on the couch in a more relaxed way. One day I noticed that he wasn't turned toward me but was looking at a watercolor on the wall opposite. He began to muse about that blue-and-gray painting, its undefined mood. Was it about to storm or about to clear? Who defined the mood of the painting, the painter or the viewer? Strikingly, Samuel didn't ask me to answer but went on to talk about a memory of his own internal storminess on vacations with his family. This was the first session in which Samuel moved to interior space without turning to me to articulate things for him.

Where interactive therapeutic process had pulled Samuel away from himself, silence created a protective buffer between us. It wasn't until later that this mostly self-analytic work moved into the relational arena and Samuel began to explore his reactions to others, including me.

Both interior and relational (articulated) aspects of analytic process were engaged here. Within intersubjective space, Samuel and I identified the element of reenactment (of his parents' omniscience) as it played out between us. Yet Samuel couldn't use that understanding to establish a sense of interiority; he first needed to temporarily sequester himself from the dyadic arena.

## Interiority and the developing containing function

Some people struggle less with articulating emotional process than with tolerating it in the absence of a responsive, soothing other. Interpersonal contact contains anxiety by pulling the person away from the self; transference exploration and relational dialogue tend to obscure this difficulty with self-regulation.

By profession a painter, Martha revealed herself to be an intuitive relationalist who kept our interaction at the center of the therapeutic dialogue. Martha insisted that I acknowledge my impact on her, confronting me with evidence of my inconsistency or other breaches; at other moments, she more shyly expressed warm feelings toward me.

Martha was highly attuned to her impact on me. Sensitive to my experience of her, Martha noted (accurately) that I enjoyed the intensity of our involvement but found it difficult to be constantly scrutinized. Her interest in my subjectivity made sense given childhood experiences with self-involved, critical young parents who left her feeling both alone and inadequate. With me, Martha both rediscovered and attempted to redress that aloneness. It was especially important to her that I acknowledge my hurtful impact; in so doing, I was different from her parents, who couldn't tolerate her negative feelings. Yet, I was also like her mother—I left just when she needed me, turning my attention to another patient or to my personal life.

Ironically, then, mutual engagement pulled Martha away from herself. She could process and master feelings of rejection, vulnerability, envy, and rage only when I named and actively contained her experience. Camouflaged by our rich interaction was Martha's difficulty tolerating her own insideness and the aloneness accompanying it. Her feelings overwhelmed and frightened her; she became frantic until she found an empathic listener. It was Martha's tolerance for interior experience that was limited; she couldn't live *in* her feelings without a validating other who responded to her with recognition.

Shortly before the summer break, Martha became silent for the first time in our work together. Although she lay quietly on the couch, the power of her feelings was palpably expressed in her face and body language. The emotional richness of that silence was such that I didn't want to break into it, although I didn't altogether understand its meaning. Quite atypically, we remained silent for the rest of the session. When I indicated that our time was up, Martha sat up, looked at me with great intensity, and, uncharacteristically, said "Thank you" as she left. Martha didn't refer to that session again but seemed to approach our separation with less anxiety than usual. And though I wanted to ask her about that silent session, I sensed that I shouldn't.

When we resumed in the fall, Martha began and ended many sessions with periods of silence—up to about ten minutes in length. Occasionally, I've asked her about her experience of silence. She says she needs to be quiet with me, that it feels good to be with me in her feelings. She usually says little else about it.

Martha uses silence to create moments of contained affective resiliency. Of course, I implicitly represent a silent witness; she feels alone in my presence rather than absolutely alone. This quiet therapeutic space seems to support a deepening level of genuine, less anxious connectedness and a gradual lessening of Martha's reliance on me for affect regulation. Now she brings me her experience, sometimes partially processed, and works with me on its meanings rather than needing me to contain it for her.

Should I have inquired about the meaning of these silences with Samuel and Martha? Certainly I wanted to. But if my patient needs an emotional experience to be hers alone, that kind of dialogue, while useful on one level, masks a more essential issue. It wasn't until Samuel and Martha solidified their experience of insideness that I could do so without reenacting this core difficulty.

I use these vignettes to illustrate holding's function with people whose central difficulties involve affect articulation and affect regulation (see Ruth Stein's (2008) principle of affect sparing). But even people who ordinarily can contact and sustain interior experience sometimes need this kind of holding. There are moments when the very act of putting our subjective process into words dilutes it and depletes it of texture and richness. We guard what's ours and what's private *not* because we're afraid of the other's failure but because at that moment, our interiority is more valuable than intersubjective exchange. The unknown, uncommunicated aspect of human experience is, as Winnicott noted, ubiquitous. For our patients and for ourselves.

## Beyond dependence

While neither Samuel nor Martha was intensely dependent on me, the affective color of our sessions was mostly reflective and soft. Lest I leave you thinking that holding always organizes around vulnerability, though, I want to underscore that there are times when patients need us to hold many other kinds of affect states—including anger, ruthlessness, and self-involvement. In all these emotional situations, holding means accepting—rather than challenging, interpreting, or countering—our patient's experience while bracketing our subjectivity as much as we can (see Slochower, 1996c and 2014d, for clinical examples).

Holding narcissism means trying to contain our impatience and our wish to do "real" analytic work. It means tolerating how little seems to be happening without interpreting the defensive function of a patient's self-involvement or concreteness *or* explicitly introducing myself (my ideas or my feelings). Holding hate or contempt means accepting a patient's negative feelings without interpreting or challenging them. I once responded to a hateful patient who was unremittingly nasty and attacking by saying, in all seriousness, "You really have yourself a lousy analyst" (see the case of Karen in Slochower, 1992). Said in a tough tone, I implicitly confirmed Karen's experience of me *and* communicated that I'm resilient enough to survive her attack without retaliating (Winnicott, 1971), although I am, indeed, a bit irritated (as she expects me to be).

Across a multiplicity of clinical situations then, holding means containing the wish to name and explore my patient's impact on me. It also means refraining from interpreting the reenactment (for the moment), or defending myself (Davies & Frawley, 1994; Grand, 2000, 2010). Holding may help a patient contact painful feelings such as rage, self-loathing, longing, and so on. At other times, it helps her move out of a flooded emotional state. But whatever its shape, holding creates a clinical/theoretical envelope within which I function more like a subjective than a "real" object.

The holding metaphor pulls us to partially set aside the parental/analytic protest ("Hey, wait a minute. What about me? Mothers/analysts are people too"). So, holding requires a lot of self-holding on the analyst's part. Further, working this way isn't fun or easy: It can feel oppressive, limiting, can leave us thinking we're not doing enough work or that we're constantly holding our breath, staying too still, tracking our patient too closely (note that I'm pointing to the useful edge of self-holding, in contrast to Winnicott's idea that self-holding always represents a false self function).

To what extent does the holding metaphor apply to contemporary work? We don't often see the kind of regression Winnicott and his colleagues described. Even my analytic patients rarely come more than three times weekly. To some extent, the contemporary context pulls against a full regression and may limit a patient's need for holding (or capacity to use therapeutic space in that way). Nevertheless I suspect that we hold, albeit more subtly today than in earlier analytic times. In Chapter 2, I revisit the holding theme from a contemporary perspective, explore holding's limits, deconstruct the holding-expressivity binary, and describe how underlying shame dynamics intensify people's need for holding.

# Chapter 2

## Revisiting the maternal metaphor

### A long view

I began writing about holding in the early 1990s, a time when many relationalists were vociferously critiquing developmental tilt models. *Holding and Psychoanalysis* (1996c, 2014c) elaborates on the therapeutic power of holding in a range of clinical situations and reformulates the role of the analyst's subjectivity in it. Underscoring holding's co-constructed element, I explored the patient's participation in the bracketing process that's central to relational holding. Here I take a second look at the holding theme from a contemporary perspective.

### Revisiting the holding-mutuality binary

The holding theme was traditionally viewed as a way of working that precludes interpretation, confrontation, or the joint analysis of enactments. Indeed, holding and mutuality are typically described as a polarity characterized by nondisclosure on one end and full disclosure on the other.

But it's a false dichotomy: Despite our best attempts at containment, aspects of our personhood—its dimensionality and its limits—leak into therapeutic space. It's inevitable; we cannot *not* show ourselves. Besides which, we show plenty of ourselves by virtue of how and when we hold.

Further, the other end of this polarity is equally elusive. Even when we aim for full disclosure and ongoing mutual exploration, we never quite get there. Nor, I believe, should we. Full disclosure is impossible (because we analysts have our own unconscious experience). It's also undesirable. No matter how much we value intersubjectivity, there will always be information and feelings that we choose not to tell because of our wish for privacy and/or because it's too disruptive, too disturbing, or too hurtful to do otherwise. We choose (partially unconsciously) what we try to bracket (contain and study) and what we express based on a mixture of our patient's and our

DOI: 10.4324/9781032691534-4

own needs, wishes, and anxieties, along with our clinical ideas about what's therapeutic and what's not. I'm convinced this is true, no matter where we sit on the restraint-expressivity continuum.

Psychoanalytic theories are most often formulated in opposition to clashing ones, an ongoing series of correctives that easily become pendulum swings. Early relational writing corrected the excesses of hierarchical, one-person, drive-based theories (Greenberg & Mitchell, 1983). My work on holding rebalanced that corrective in a third direction by detailing the limits of mutuality. It provoked its own reaction, and in the 1990s, Bass (1996) and I had a lively argument about whether it's possible to hold, rather than to hold back or hold on; that is, whether holding obfuscates what we prefer not to see. And, inevitably, it does: First, we're always holding something back, no matter how little we intentionally hold; second, even when we're trying to hold, we're also expressing aspects of our subjectivity. This chapter moves past the holding-expressivity polarity and explores their interpenetration.

## Developmental metaphors in 2023

Relational thinking has evolved. Influenced by Loewald, the attachment theorists, Benjamin, and, perhaps, my own position, Mitchell's later work addressed the role of early relational dynamics in analytic experience. Although he never explicitly privileged the patient's baby needs, he no longer insisted on patient-as-adult. In *Relationality* (2000), Mitchell articulated a layered vision of an adult influenced by a range of modalities, some of which originate in infancy. Rather than viewing adult and baby states as a binary (needy baby vs. mature adult), we've come to recognize that the adult moves fluidly between adult, child, and baby states.

We've also moved away from schematic developmental models and notions of a fixed and sequential growth process. Those formulations collide with theories of nonlinear movement and multiple self-states (Bromberg, 1991; Corbett, 2008; Davies & Frawley, 1994; Goldner, 1991; Harris, 2009; Mitchell, 1993). But theories of multiplicity don't negate the presence of baby states within analytic process—they make room for them. We don't have to choose between baby and grown-up; even when our patient feels like an adult, she has the capacity—perhaps disavowed, perhaps not—to access and temporarily move into a baby state. And vice versa (Slochower, 2017a, 2018a).

Contemporary views of the relational baby emerge not out of idealized visions of mother and baby, but from infant research findings. This baby is actively engaged with the (m)other; she's not the passive recipient of good-enough (or not good-enough) parental care. She's a different, more active kind of baby, reactive to *and* a participant in Mother's own pulls and pushes. Still, the legacy of those early attachment patterns can be found in analytic space because adult distress sometimes carries the shadow of that baby.

Over the last decade, other theoretical strands, too many to catalog here, have entered the developmental conversation (see Seligman, 2003). Pivotal has been the contribution of attachment research and dynamic systems theories that delineate the processes underlying self-regulatory, comfort-seeking, and mutual regulatory interactive patterns (e.g., Ainsworth, 1969; Beebe & Lachmann, 1994, 1998; Beebe, Lachmann, Markese, & Bahrick, 2012; Hesse & Main, 2000; Stolorow, 1997). Their work expands our understanding of what's behind the global holding metaphor and unpacks its nonverbal dimension.

As we invite baby states back into the consulting room, we address the baby's legacy, if not the baby herself, while also exploring the mother's (and analyst's) complex role in co-shaping these patterns. I'd add that the analyst's own babyhood is implicated here; at moments, there may be *two* babies in the consulting room. The analyst's early regulatory patterns are activated along with—and in reaction to—the patient's.

Some of us relationalists—including Benjamin (1988, 1995a), Bromberg (1998), Davies (1994, 1998), Grand (2000), Harris (2009), Warshaw (1992), and—use implicit developmental models. But writers including Hoffman (2009) and D. B. Stern (1997), who are interested not in developmental patterns but in interactive ones, also echo aspects of these themes.

The need for moments of attuned responsiveness emerges across our lifetime, however grown-up, "separated," or reflective we are (see Ogden's (1986, 1989) idea of simultaneous but shifting affective modalities). And this need isn't limited to patients with a history of massive early trauma; almost all of my patients (and all of us analysts) have moments when that "no longer baby" is as palpable as our own parental identification and reparative fantasy. Like my Wall Street patient who phoned me in a panic because something his wife said made him feel that the sky was falling. For the first time in his remembered life, he had someone to call; I became, for a moment, a soothing presence, someone who could receive his distress, accept rather than counter it without also becoming dysregulated. He felt held, and slowly calmed down enough to think about what he was feeling. Together we enacted a version of the parental metaphor. But just for that moment.

It's the concrete that gets us into trouble: When we insist that the patient *is* a baby *or* insist that she's an adult capable of mutuality, we skip over the interpenetrating nature of baby and grown-up self-states and pull for one or the other in a way that may feel "as if" or pseudo. Either can be shaming of the patient. The patient seen as baby may feel shame over her envy or hate; the patient seen as an adult may feel shame over her vulnerability and merger longings.

## Holding's dynamic function: Buffering shame states

Holding alludes to the enacted reparative element, a sort of corrective emotional experience. We don't call it corrective in Alexander's (1950) sense when we hold or when we function as a new object, but we're doing something awfully close to that by helping create antidotes to toxic internalized object experiences and particularly shame states.

When we hold, we bear witness to our patient's experience without challenging it; we privilege her perspective on herself and allow it to unfold, received but not altered. This kind of therapeutic process is especially mutative for shame-prone individuals (Bromberg, 1998; Morrison, 1989; Orange, 2008). Shame, often organized around a sense of exposure to an unfriendly, critical eye, is activated by the feeling of being seen from the outside, looked "at," looked down upon. Holding buffers shame because the experience of affective attunement—however it's configured—creates a shield against exposure. The illusion of analytic resonance remains unchallenged and uncomplicated; my patient feels *with* me rather than seen *by* me. Over time, the holding experience allows a scaffold to coalesce that protects her against humiliation and permits us to enter the arena of shame. Together. And eventually will allow us to move toward explicitly intersubjective work.

Over the years, I've given many examples of holding's therapeutic function in work around dependence, rage, narcissism, and ruthlessness. Although holding's function in buffering shame was implicit in some of those examples, it wasn't explicit. Here, I illustrate how holding moments organized outside the arena of the maternal metaphor can buffer shame.

Mark, an academic in his early 50s, came for analysis about a decade ago. He grew up with a contemptuous, physically abusive father and a passive, mostly absent mother who seemed not to connect to him. Mark's young adulthood was characterized by drift—from relationship to relationship and career to career. In early middle age, he met his current partner, Chris, and something about Chris's stable evenness repaired things enough for Mark to settle into a reasonably solid relationship and career, although his trauma history periodically made itself known.

Coming to me at Chris's request, Mark was defensive, argumentative, and avoidant, but also ruefully aware that his irritability was casting a pall on his relationship. As he put it, "Chris will kill me if I don't do this. But then again, I might just kill him and myself first. Metaphorically speaking only, of course." Smart and funny, yet staving off a major depression, Mark settled into a three-times-weekly treatment. He was self-reflective in an intellectualized sort of way, shifting between angry, bitter moods and a more curious and lively sense of self. He could think about his past and connect it to his choice of partner, someone with whom it was safe to get angry. Mark also noted that there had been no mother *there* to be angry with, teasingly adding that it was a good thing I had a bigger impact than my size might suggest. Mark's easy humor would become a mainstay of our work.

But mostly Mark wasn't funny—he was painfully sad and bitter. Listening to his reminiscences, I imagined this little boy's loneliness and fear as he contended with his powerful, irritable father and absent mother. Because Mark spoke so freely, I wasn't immediately aware that things went well only when I listened. When I entered the conversation actively—whether to ask a question, make a comment, or offer a tentative interpretation, when I expressed my sense of what Mark was feeling—things went less well. Mark would pause briefly and then go on speaking as if he hadn't heard me. Occasionally, he nodded before continuing, but his nod mainly felt like a way to get me to shut up. When I persisted, Mark changed the subject, usually to something external to us both. When he described especially painful memories and I reacted verbally (e.g., saying, "That sounds just awful"), even making an empathic sound, he paused only briefly before either cracking a joke or altogether leaving the interior arena and launching into a description of something going on in the world. When I asked Mark whether what I had said bothered him, he ignored my question, sometimes cracked another joke, but always moved into a third space. Mostly that third space involved the political scene and his sophisticated analysis of it. Although aware of its defensive function, I found myself engrossed by Mark's astute (and resonant) political perspective and amused by his joke telling.

Yet I also sensed we were using these conversations as a way out of the self-conscious state into which Mark feared he would fall—or already had fallen. He needed to keep himself (and us) at a distance, and although anxieties about merger probably underlaid this need, it seemed impossible to name. And so, when the moment seemed as right as it ever was, I gently tried to name some of this. Mark grew very still on the couch. Nodding, he flushed intensely but remained silent. Waiting a bit, I said even more gently that I thought I had just embarrassed him, that being seen or understood by me felt painfully exposing. After a pause, Mark nodded and said, almost in a whisper, "Please don't." Sensing that he couldn't say more, I said only "I'll try." And I did. Mostly.

Mark tolerated engaging with me only when our bond stayed light and humorous. I struggled to honor that—to hold him—by giving him space and containing my feelings, especially my resonant sadness with Mark's pain, pain he thinly veiled with humor. My explicitly empathizing with his sadness intensified Mark's shame and derailed the protected space in which he dwelled. And so, Mark undertook a kind of self-analysis to which I was witness more than participant.

It was another full year before Mark cried in my office and longer still before he allowed himself to ask for my input, let alone my caring. But, in time, all of that came about, and gradually Mark's "self-analysis" became a dyadic one. With a decade of work behind us, we're getting close to being done, and spoke recently about the idea of terminating.

Still, Mark's skittishness remains a clear and present thread. Now, though, he announces his intensifying defensiveness with a joke: "OK, enough of your thoughts. I'm taking a sharp left turn," turning away from himself and into left-wing politics. Smart, funny, interesting, he banters, and I banter back. We laugh, occasionally we debate a bit. It's fun for us both.

Ordinarily, I don't connect humor with holding. Humor is a register that feels far more spontaneous; it embodies so much of one's subjectivity, so much interpenetrating affect. But I've come to think about Mark's humor and my amused response as providing a co-created holding function, albeit an atypical one. It emerges whenever Mark touches edges of his trauma history, when his sense of intactness or need for me becomes acute. Mark beats a quick retreat from both into the land of humor, into his version of Jon Stewart's *The Daily Show*, a TV show we both love. Mark's jokes get me to laugh and rebalance things between us because as I do, he experiences aspects of his own aliveness while also symbolically enlivening his deadened, depressed mother. Shared humor serves as a buffer against the double threats of humiliating exposure in the face of an unresponsive object and assault, both precipitants of shame states.

But I don't want to leave you with the impression that holding was all that happened in Mark's treatment. It wasn't. We did lots of work that had nothing to do with holding. I sometimes spoke confrontationally to Mark about aspects of my difficult experience of him, about his edginess and sarcasm. There were reenactments as well, times when I failed Mark in just the way he needed me not to fail. All of these had their own therapeutic—and counter-therapeutic—effects. We struggled and did some negotiating (S. A. Pizer, 1998). I could, in fact, write a whole paper on the enactments and negotiations in Mark's treatment. But because here I'm thinking about babies, I'm tilting things the other way and underscoring the backdrop against which all this juicier stuff took place. Like Sandler's (1960) background of safety, our laughter was the linchpin around which the rest was organized. Though perhaps some of you would say that enactments were the linchpin and holding the thing that killed time between them (Spezzano, 1998).

Mark's intense vulnerability to shame states made it near impossible to name or explore them, yet they lurked at the edge of nearly everything he spoke about. And when intensely evoked, they were intensely derailing. I suspect that my laughter, via processes of interpretive action (Ogden, 1994), helped Mark access and sustain a non-humiliated self-state at moments of acute shame. Recently he put words to this: "Sometimes I thought I was a pathetic, slobbery wimp. Someone everyone would point at and laugh at. So instead, I got you to laugh, and when you did, I refound another part of me. And I no longer felt ashamed." Only now, with an end in sight, are we explicitly working with these shame dynamics—essential work, but elusive outside the holding experience.

For patients such as Mark, and sometimes for the analyst as well (Stein, 1997), shame is evoked by the exposure of baby needs. For others, though, shame is triggered by feelings including anger, desire, or greed. And, ironically, sometimes it's the holding experience itself that evokes shame. I imagine you won't be surprised to hear that in the context of our tentative exploration of shame Mark once said, "I need not to need you to be any particular way with me. If I feel your support, I feel ashamed of the fact that I want it. It has to be okay for you to be however you are being. And it's not." At that point in our work, there was no evading shame.

The therapeutic power of witnessing has been the subject of writing on major trauma (Boulanger, 2007; Gerson, 2009; Grand, 2000, 2010; Harris, 2009; Laub, 1992; Laub & Auerhahn, 1993; Laub & Podell, 1995; Rosenblum, 2009). This literature underscores witnessing's reparative impact in work with Holocaust survivors and other victims of the unspeakable. Yet I think it's also true that all of our patients—and all of us—have been traumatized insofar as we've experienced nonrecognition in moments of acute need (D. B. Stern, 2009).

## Holding and its underbelly

Holding, like many Winnicottian concepts, invites overuse, indeed, mis-use. The construct can be too schematic, over-read, bled of its therapeutic usefulness. Nearly any intervention can be justified as holding, supporting a regression, expanding transitional space—in fact, it's an idea that can be invoked to describe almost anything we do other than actively confront or piercingly interpret. Holding can also be used to justify inaction. I've heard analysts describe having held a patient by literally giving her a transitional object—as if anyone but the patient can imbue the concrete with transition-ality. A supervisee once described how he "held" his patient by remaining impassive when shown a photo of the patient's beautiful girlfriend. I'd say he was being competitively withholding and had called his behavior "hold-ing" to rationalize.

In a similar way, holding a regression to dependence has mostly lost its original meaning as an organized response to a patient by an analyst capa-ble of receiving and containing intense affect states without collapsing or retaliating. Too often, holding is conflated with the notion of regression, a return to earlier, "immature" modes of relating, a blueprint for a kind of straight-line therapeutic process in which we repair the baby.

But there was never simply a baby/patient in the consulting room. Older children—and we adults—sometimes need holding too, sometimes from within a much younger self-state, sometimes from a very adult but very vul-nerable self-state. I recently had a long conversation with someone experi-encing a frightening medical crisis. In her own language, she told me how held she felt by people's capacity to meet her where she was emotionally, even though she hadn't asked. There's nothing infantile about that. It's just human.

## The takeaway

Baby and child metaphors embody the phenomenological reality of these states while temporarily ignoring the other actuality, that of patient-as-adult. I think we can, finally, take both for granted. And although these developmental metaphors have been critiqued for their idealization of both the analytic and therapeutic function, this critique can be leveled at any therapeutic model: Whether we think about patients' needs for confrontation, authenticity, mutuality, selfobject experiences, or recognition, we idealize something.

Our ideal represents our wish, and often also our need, to heal, to change, to engage, to do something useful. Of course, our personhood limits our capacity to meet that ideal, and confronts us with what I've called a psychoanalytic collision (Slochower, 2006c, 2014b, 2015b). Collisions emerge, independent of our theoretical allegiance, out of the space between our professional ideal and the actuality of our human fallibility.

In fact, my writing has confronted me with another collision: Despite my immersion in the holding theme, I rarely work like a Winnicottian. I usually play it pretty straight; that is, I try to find a way to articulate what I'm thinking and why, and I "hold back" very little. Indeed, many of my analyst patients have pointed out (often—but not always—affectionately) that I don't seem like a holding analyst to them; I'm more often described as someone who "calls a spade a spade," albeit nicely. Further, much of me is embedded *within* the holding metaphor, reflected in the ways I try to hold.

Over time, I've become more relaxed, more expressive of my subjectivity. A bit less cautious. Yet with many patients, exploration, interpretation, confrontation, and reenactment all coexist with a background awareness of their vulnerability to shame states and need for holding. So, in a way, I hold even when I push. All of this, of course, gets experienced and expressed in a range of ways (good and bad) by different patients.

So, to get back to the beginning: There's no simple baby—or adult—in the consulting room because both members of the dyad move from moment to moment, imperceptibly and unconsciously, toward and away from mutuality. In this process, they contact, enact, and perhaps meet the needs of these baby and child self-states, for better and for worse.

We don't have to abandon the idea of a psychoanalytic baby because it can, in fact, swim in relational bathwater (Seligman, 2012)—bathwater that includes an analyst who holds and who fails to hold, who's mostly, but not always, capable of self-reflectivity, who has access to her own baby self-states and sometimes mixes it up with her patient. The developmental trajectory, such as it is, has so many bumps and reversals that it would be absurd to call it linear. Still, the notion of progression from a world dominated by the experience of a single subject to one characterized by interpenetrating subjectivities and mutuality—a shifting, rather than a linear progression—remains appealing. En route to that goal, we hold, each in our own idiosyncratic way, whatever word we use to describe it.

In chapters 3, 4, and 5 I move beyond relational holding to explore and critique other clinical ideas that were rejected by early relational thinking. I begin with the notion of resistance.

# Chapter 3

# Resist this

Relational analysts tend to be resistant to talking about resistance. There are many reasons for this, some theoretical and some not. From a theoretical perspective, the concept seems too classically one-person, too certain, too pre-postmodern. It resides too far outside the realm of enactment, an arena at the center of therapeutic action. But there are also personal reasons for avoiding the concept. Many of us resist the term resistance because we want to avoid experiencing the countertransference it evokes. It's not pleasant to think, much less write, about treatment moments characterized by the R word. I don't like how I feel about myself and my patient when I'm thinking she's resistant. The word labels, even blames her. It polarizes the dyad and closes down reflective space.

In earlier psychoanalytic times, the concept figured large in our theorizing. A patient's defensive response to interpretations was evidence of a dynamically driven resistance, beneath which lay an unconscious evasion of the anxiety, aggression, guilt, or shame that the interpretation evoked (e.g., Adler & Bachant, 1998; Freud, 1896; Kernberg, 1974; Klein, 1975; Kohut, 1971, 1977; Rangell, 1983). Used well, these kinds of dynamic formulations helped us by identifying our patient's self-protective investment in keeping things as they were. They clarified underlying anxieties and allowed us to move more deeply into what was frightening, unknown, or disavowed.

But used badly, the concept didn't help at all. "Resistance" could too easily be engaged to reassert the validity of our dynamic understanding ("I'm right, you're just resisting accepting a painful truth"). Rather than creating a feeling of dyadic linkage, we used it to pull away from our patient: "My patient is . . . difficult/negative/massively defensive/not suitable for analysis. Nothing links us."

DOI: 10.4324/9781032691534-5

Even when we avoided othering our resistant patient, we remained the purveyor of truth, knowledge, and dynamic accuracy. Our interpretation may have been maladroit or excessively penetrating, but we rarely concluded that we had simply been wrong. We had been guilty, at worst, of crappy timing.

We've come a long way since then, and I think this is true whatever the particulars of our particular theory. Across Freudian, interpersonal, relational, self psychology, and other orientations, we've moved past the impasse that early conceptualizations of resistance invited. We're less likely to assume we simply have it right and less likely to blame patients when they reject what we say. Many of us agree on one "fact"—that there are no facts, outside the realm of our patient's subjective experience. Who's to say that we really know what's going on? Or that it's our patient who's resisting our "correct" interpretation? Perhaps we're the one resisting understanding something that's true for our patient, subjectively speaking. Might our countertransference be occluding that understanding? Is a mutual resistance at play? Or might we unconsciously be colluding with our patient to stay away from what's hot by focusing on something else?

By examining the relational dynamics embedded in what feels like resistance, we move beyond the power struggle/conflict element that early conceptualizations of the concept invited. We create more room within which to consider our impact and the enactment that's obscured by the resistant element (e.g., Bromberg, 2006; Hoffman, 1991; Renik, 1995). Underneath what looks like a power struggle may lie a desperate attempt at self-stabilization (Ainsworth, 1969; Beebe & Lachmann, 1994, p. 2002; Hesse & Main, 2000; Stolorow, 1997). Yes, resistance is a defense, but it's a defense conceptualized in urgent terms: Our patient resists our input because we've threatened to precipitate disorganization or dissociation. This perspective allows us to examine ourselves rather than blame our patient.

## What about our own resistance?

It's not only our patients who become resistant when threatened. When our interpretations fail repeatedly, when we're regularly stymied or chronically fall flat, we can be tempted to offload our frustration by invoking the "resistant" label ("There's nothing wrong with what I'm doing/saying; you're resistant/defensive/impossible"). We turn to a slightly more sophisticated version of the third grader's glue-and-rubber refrain: "I'm rubber, you're glue, what you say to me bounces back to you." Our conceptualization becomes its own resistance; we reassert its validity in an unconscious attempt to evade the inadequacy or frustration that would surface were we to recognize that we're wrong. Or, catapulted into hopelessness, we blame our patient, decide that she's concrete, lacks a capacity for symbolic process. We resist remaining in the clinical moment and pull back or pull out. We give up, explicitly or secretly. Both our patient's and our own reflective space collapse.

But even if we succeed in offloading our discomfort by blaming our patient, we're stuck with the feelings simultaneously evoked. We don't like feeling the way we do. We don't like finger pointing. These moments of impasse are as much of our own making as they are our patient's, but our frustration and helplessness make it extraordinarily difficult to query our participation in them.

How and why are we so invested in what we're saying? How anxious, angry, or frustrated are we feeling? What if we have it wrong? What if we've been too intrusively right? And what's at stake for us? Do we need our patient to appreciate what we're saying because it validates our competence or disconfirms a disturbing sense of inadequacy? Because it reassures us of our importance to her? What are we trying to prove to ourselves? To her?

Today we're less likely to locate resistance squarely in the patient; instead, we ask ourselves whether a jointly reenacted element is at play. Have we repeated a sticky family dynamic—were we too certain, too insistent? Did our interpretation feel like a symbolic assault to be evaded at all costs? We also more easily consider the possibility that, rather than being too right, we might, in fact, simply be wrong.

Implicit in this shift is a recognition that what looks like resistance may mask underlying trauma dynamics. It's not merely that our interpretation is anxiety-arousing; what we said—and/or how we said it—repeated an early experience of overwhelm, attack, or annihilation. By identifying the traumatic impact of our interpretation, we step back from our own certainty and the power struggle it precipitated. We soften our tone, choose our words more carefully, work harder to sustain a sense of connection. We're less likely to plunge headlong into what's difficult or issue confrontational interpretations. We walk softly as we try to find a way forward.

## Entering the resistant moment

This way of conceptualizing resistance doesn't have a linear relationship to what we do in the clinical interaction, of course; each of us enters these moments in our own way. Here's mine: When I sense my patient's growing defensiveness, I offer a kind of forewarning before entering the therapeutic dialogue. That forewarning is embedded in tentativeness, itself an attempt at empathic resonance. I might say, "This is going to be hard to hear." Or "I want to float something difficult by you. I could be wrong but . . ." These kinds of acknowledgments can help soften the inherent asymmetry of the moment and mitigate my patient's experience of me as an "outside" threat or adversary.

Sometimes this helps. It creates just enough space for my patient to hear me. She may agree, argue, or correct me, but we're in conversation around her experience and that dialogue helps us shift out of a stalemate. But sometimes neither solid analytic theory nor all the tact in the world helps. No matter how carefully we rethink the clinical moment, find gentler ways to move, or address our contribution to a resistant moment, we get pushback. Our patient ignores or rejects every therapeutic offering; she seems impenetrable, hostile, or shut down, and we find ourselves in more of a chronic power struggle than an analytic dialogue.

My response to this kind of impasse is to turn away from content and instead name my patient's reaction to what I said while ignoring the content that got us there. Addressing its emotional impact, I implicitly take responsibility for her emotional experience. I might say "I'm thinking that I've made you feel pretty mad"; "I suspect I've hurt your feelings"; or "I have a hunch that what I just said bothered you."

It's my way to make statements like "I'm thinking you're mad" rather than asking a direct question like "Are you mad?" A statement doesn't require a response and so puts my patient less on the spot; it allows her to, if need be, ignore me. I also don't address the content that angered or hurt but instead shift *toward* her; I name what I suspect she feels about what I said. This more indirect approach softens the space between us and expands things in a less confrontational way. Even if I'm wrong, she may feel relieved by the effort at recognition my comment embodies.

This is, in a sense, an enacted repair; it temporarily suspends analytic inquiry with the aim of shifting us out of the resistant impasse. But for a repair to take place, my patient must be able to tolerate the awareness that I've disturbed things—i.e., that my impact on her was considerable. And some people can't bear the implicit and subjectively shameful exposure my acknowledgment evokes. Saying that I've hurt or insulted underscores her vulnerability, and that awareness is unbearable.

In these moments, I move back a bit and address things from a greater interpersonal distance while simultaneously assuming responsibility for what's going on. Staying outside the arena of "us," never explicitly identifying her vulnerability, I appropriate responsibility for my patient's distress without directly speaking to her feelings. I might say "I think I just screwed up" rather than "I bet you're upset with me." Saying things indirectly may be face-saving for someone who's desperately trying to negate her sensitivity to my impact.

Here's an illustration: Sally, overburdened by work responsibilities and the demands of extended family, experiences herself as the finger in the dike, the one who must always save the day. Sally's core identification is as victim—over extended, exploited, and used, endlessly putting out fires set by others. This way of living is exhausting and angering, and Sally shifts between states of agitated depression and weeping ("I can't believe all this is happening. It's all on me to fix. There's no room for me in my life"). Occasionally Sally's distress is interrupted by flashes of rage at those who need her and those who fail her ("Once again, my sister was unavailable, I had to take my mom back to the ER in the middle of the night, no one else would do it").

Sally volleys between alarm and an angry sense of victimization. Despite her capacity for symbolic thinking in other arenas, Sally cannot reflect on any of this. She moves from crisis to crisis, chronically dysregulated and unable to examine herself. Sally cannot mentalize, deepen interior access, or engage in affect regulation. Acutely vulnerable to a "done to" self-state (Benjamin, 2017), Sally too often feels exploited and mistreated.

I've got some hunches about why. I suspect that this victim state has origins in Sally's identification with her parents' trauma history, an identification that left her longing for recognition. When I empathize with Sally and refrain from questioning or interpreting anything, things go well; Sally feels understood, even grateful. Analysis is a safe haven, a place where she can unload and have her experience validated. But despite my hope that this holding space would help Sally look at herself, it hasn't. Sally reacts catastrophically to even minor crises. By the end of most sessions, I feel worn down, frustrated—at times, hopeless.

I've tried everything I can think of. I've said things such as "I'm thinking that taking a chance on saying 'no' would be really scary"; or "Maybe there's a way that being indispensable is important." I've tried to explore the origin of Sally's victim stance, saying "You so desperately wanted to save your parents, to relieve their suffering"; "I think you've felt overburdened all your life, but it was never possible to protest, much less get angry about it"; "You feel as alone as your mother must have."

But while my dynamic understanding of all this helps me hold myself, it doesn't seem to help Sally. Letting her in on my experience of her or asking her to think about where the other person might have been coming from also hasn't shifted things. Sally sometimes becomes defensive when I offer an interpretation or name my reaction to her, but more often she simply ignores me and persistently returns to reality. Yes, her parents were chronically overburdened and assaulted by life. That's why it's so important to her to take responsibility for her family, but really, she has no choice. If she isn't at the center of the action, everything collapses. Her life is an ongoing exercise in crisis management. Why can't I understand that there's nothing more to it?

Sally's dramatic tone, wild tears, and helpless shrugs leave me feeling less empathic than annoyed. Sometimes I want to roll my eyes. When my frustration gets too much for me, I push and get concrete. Once, I floated the idea that treating her partner as incapable might exacerbate the partner's helplessness. Did Sally need to be the only responsible one because there hadn't been anyone to count on at home? Sally nodded. Hopeful, I continued: What would happen if she had her partner take over the next project and stuck to her plan to take a day off from work? Cautiously Sally mused it would be wonderful to get to a painting class. Maybe she'd try it.

Oy! How wrong I was! Sally came into the next session in a bitter fury. She had taken my implicit advice, delegated the project to her partner and taken the day off. And what happened? Her partner screwed everything up. Trying to repair things, Sally hadn't slept in more than 36 hours. I had been naïve to think anyone else could be counted on.

Feeling bad, both about having given such non analytic advice and that the advice I gave had made things worse, I tried to regroup. Turning to process, I named Sally's anger at me for getting it wrong and tried to bracket my sense that Sally had participated in sustaining this dynamic: "I really messed things up. I thought I knew better but I didn't get it. I misread the situation by encouraging you to step back. You're desperately trying to keep your life going, to manage the loneliness and fear of being the only one. No wonder you're pissed and upset."

Sally nodded and softened. "Now you understand. I know you're trying to help me have a life of my own, but you keep thinking there's a psychological element to what's going on. There's not, I'm just describing reality."

By moving from content to process, by appropriating responsibility for my failure and refraining from addressing Sally's participation in it or the reenactment it embodied, the impasse between us gave way and we went on. Had something therapeutic happened? Or had I merely joined Sally's resistance and perpetuated our stalemate?

With some people, acknowledging our hurtfulness or empathic failure softens the power struggle inherent in the implied argument resistance involves ("Why aren't you seeing this my way?"). Often, though certainly not always, this creates a moment of meeting (D. N. Stern, 2004). We return to content, to what we said that was derailing and why. But something else happens that's more important: A window opens into the micro-impasse that has plagued our patient (and perhaps plagued us too) over time.

But not with Sally, who remains rigidly defensive and resistant to self-examination. I know my frustration leaks, but Sally seems not to react. When I name this, she rolls her eyes or sighs and quickly changes the subject. When I refrain from addressing this dynamic, I worry that I'm colluding, furthering Sally's defensiveness and tendency to externalize. But when I try to unpack the issues driving her raging self-sacrifice or query what's going on between us, Sally is superficially cooperative but then collapses into angry misery, feeling abandoned and hopeless. When I talk about her collapse, Sally bitterly tells me that I don't get it and am failing her. Sally isn't interested in exploring her own dynamics or what goes on between us. Therapy is her only safe space; she needs me to understand her, period.

Theoretically, I think I get it. Sally's insistently angry suffering serves a central dynamic function—it keeps the other on the hook. By declaring that the emperor has no clothes, Sally points to their indifference and calls it out. Simultaneously enacting her sense of victimhood and demanding it be repaired, Sally temporarily undoes a lifetime of nonrecognition. Her apparent intransigence represents a thin covering for a trauma state that precludes access to agency. Sally cannot allow me to offer her anything without again rendering herself a passive victim. Yet this leaves her (and me) utterly stuck.

I suspect we've all worked with people like Sally, people whose resistance—whatever we call it—daunts us. Not momentarily, but chronically.

Our clinical skill comes to naught; our interpretive acumen falls on deaf ears; confrontations either are evaded or precipitate crises and/or abrupt terminations. Attempts to locate things intersubjectively by addressing the reenacted element fall flat or worse. Explicit expressions of our subjectivity/countertransference evoke irritation/fury. Or are ignored.

Sometimes it's our own myopia that occludes. Sometimes it's our conceptual or emotional cluelessness or rigidity, our resistance to recognizing our participation in a reenactment, that stalls things. Here, it's we who need to go back to go because it's we who have been getting in the way. But I don't think it's always about us, our character style, interpersonal clumsiness, dynamic blind spot, or theoretical insistence. Despite the possibility that the impasse we're experiencing reflects our own anxieties or resistances, I'm convinced that sometimes it really is our patient who's resistant.

Certainly, we don't all respond to resistant dynamics in identical ways. Some of us are better at finding a way around an impasse than others. Some of us are more easily pulled into power struggles or have more of a need to be right. Others react negatively/critically to a patient's helplessness and apparent lack of interest in changing. Our own character style and/or a "too good" fit between our issues and our patient's will be reflected in the intensity of our reaction.

## And then there's the individual resistant element

But we can't always ascribe resistance to what's intersubjective. There's also an individual dynamic that's sometimes carried across time and across treatment experiences, stymieing us as it did the therapist(s) who failed before we came on the scene. Haven't we all had the experience of taking on someone with a history of failed treatments, determined to do better? And while we may do better for a while, we eventually encounter the very resistant blockades we thought we could circumvent. Our referring colleague's description of this person turns out to be one we recognize all too well.

Here we encounter a new resistance, an inversion of its earlier iteration: Where classical analysts resist *not* locating resistance in the patient, relational analysts resist the obverse. Our belief in the overarching intersubjective element makes us skeptical of the possibility that some things reside outside the realm of the dyadic.

Might this be an overcorrection?

I'd like to invite the idea of the difficult patient—separate from the difficult dyad—back into relational space. To make room for the possibility that there are people with whom we get stuck, not because we're caught up in a reenactment, not because of our own difficult character structure, but because of our patient's particular way of being in the world. Her underlying structure blocks us despite our good enough intuition, capacity for empathy, and theoretical conceptualization. She's "difficult," and may even tell us that her friends and colleagues know this about her. She's "gone through" many analysts, all of whom failed. Even when we assiduously address the co-constructed, reenacted edge of that difficulty, the resistance remains, impervious to good interpretations, powerful moments of self-disclosure, or confrontation. Certainly, calling such people character disordered, concrete, or perseverative doesn't help. The labels pathologize rather than clarify. But her immovability remains.

And so, I'd like to go back to the beginning, to the assumption that we should always approach resistance by aiming to open things up and work them through. What if we turn the concept of resistance on its head and consider the therapeutic possibility inherent *in it*? Could this open another point of clinical entrée, one focused on resistance's potential rather than its function as a clinical obstacle?

I'm suggesting that there are times when resistance uninterpreted is a good thing, analytically speaking. When our patient's rejection of us—of our idea, suggestion, interpretation, etc., is itself mutative where working through isn't. I wonder whether our need to sustain a good-analyst feeling (Epstein, 1999) has obfuscated the clinical value of impasse unresolved.

I return to Sally. I suspect that need to assert, rather than examine, her victim stance may embody a symbolic repair. As Sally declares, indeed dramatizes her distress, she finds a witness for it and requires that the witness (me) *not* demand that she change. Sally symbolically (and literally) says no to me—no to my understanding and no to my ideas about her. She thereby delineates and sustains her boundaries so that the other's (my) power and authority neither penetrate nor overwhelm.

Sally's resistance blocks insight and stops us from working through enactments, but it also fortifies her sense of interiority and agency. It makes the space hers; it keeps me present but—unlike her parents—at a distance. I cannot influence Sally, but I can receive her experience, something that didn't happen historically.

Might Sally's resistance to self-examination be a kind of emotional "Custer's last stand" that itself contains therapeutic potential? I'm hoping, but am not yet sure, that this is what's going on. I sustain myself—mostly—because there have been some tiny shifts suggesting that things are less globally stalemated. Sally is somewhat calmer, less often very late to sessions, and cancels less frequently. She signed up for a weekly art class and makes it there about half the time. Very occasionally Sally allows me to link her early history to what's going on in the present and nods rather than ragefully rejecting my input. Recently she acknowledged that she's always angry and wishes she weren't. That felt big to me.

But there's been no seismic shift, no dramatic enactment. Too often (for me), Sally returns to an ensconced, angry, victimized state. And I remain unsure whether more global change will be possible. Will Sally's stubborn rejection of my input, her insistence that her experience is simply real and not open to examination, gradually repair a lifetime of disconfirmation? Will her "resistance" be the vehicle through which change accrues? Will Sally begin to move—albeit glacially—in the direction of reflectivity precisely because I've allowed that resistance to remain largely unchallenged?

Most clinical vignettes of this sort end with a breakthrough, often one precipitated by a dramatic enactment. But this one doesn't. I think it's important that we talk together about treatments like this one, treatments where the resistant wall remains largely unbreached. Treatments that evoke our resistance to talking (even thinking) about them because they're so undramatic, boring, flat, and frustrating.

Moments of resistance sometimes give way when we examine our investment in a particular theoretical/clinical position, our countertransference, and the intersubjective dynamics informing our patient's refusal to take in what we're doing or saying. But not always.

Must we make peace with the idea that some patients are really unable to move, no matter whom they're working with, no matter how skilled, tactful, or reflective the analyst is? To recognize that resistance is sometimes incredibly resistant to change and consider the clinical potential inherent in resistance unresolved? Must we also accept our own resistance to acknowledging the limits of our clinical capacity while simultaneously opening the door to another avenue of clinical change?

# Chapter 4

# Going too far

## Relational heroines and relational excess

Every psychoanalytic theory is organized around an implicit clinical ideal—a vision of the kind of analyst we want to be and the kind of change we hope psychoanalysis will effect. Embedded in our vision are corresponding notions of our ideal patient/process and of what's problematic.

Our ideal is often formulated in conversation (actually, in argument) with its theoretical predecessors and competitors. While those conversations can deepen and enrich our thinking, they frequently don't. Instead, they become fighting words that generate a slide toward excess by exaggerating difference and rigidifying the core principles to which we adhere. We polarize, elevating the originality of our own contribution while minimizing, stereotyping, sometimes denigrating, the position of the psychoanalytic Other whose ideals collide—or overlap excessively—with our own. Each pendulum swing seems inevitably to provoke a countermove that itself overcorrects. I think we always go a bit too far.

Perhaps it's only in hindsight that we can pause and moderate those overcorrections. Relational thinking has matured beyond our beginnings—we've got a history and so hindsight is possible. It's in this spirit that I revisit early relational theory and practice and consider where we've been, where and how we may have gone too far, and where we can go now. Whom do we aim to be in the consulting room? How do we view our patient—her potential and her limitations? What are the clinical goals of a relational analysis? And what might those goals occlude?

While this chapter focuses on relational theory, every psychoanalytic theory embodies its own ideals and is vulnerable to theoretical/clinical excess and limitations. To my knowledge, no psychoanalytic theory has addressed either from the inside out.

DOI: 10.4324/9781032691534-6

## Relational ideals

Relationalists may be theoretically diverse, but we share an implicit and relatively distinct professional ideal. It first coalesced around the value of asymmetrical mutuality and uncertainty. Emphasizing the therapeutic potential inherent in unpacking and working through what's enacted, we rejected authoritarian models and analytic visions of interpretive accuracy; we moved toward asymmetrical egalitarianism (Aron, 1991). Moderating our power and omniscience, we affirmed our patient's capacity to see us, to function as an adult in the analytic context.

Relational writers emphasized the inherently intersubjective nature of therapeutic process and the mutative potential inherent in enactment. Unformulated experience, dissociation, and shifting self-states shape analytic process for patient *and* analyst because we're implicated along with our patients. Moving away from old analytic constrictions, we found new ways to be and to use ourselves (e.g., Aron, 1999; Bass, 2001; Benjamin, 1995a, 1998; Bromberg, 1993, 1995, 1998, 2011; Davies, 1998, 2004; Davies & Frawley, 1994; Harris, 2009; Hoffman, 1991, 1998; Mitchell, 1984, 1988, 1991, 1993, 1997; D. B. Stern, 1992, 1997, 2009, 2015).

Although it isn't always acknowledged, the relational ideal was strongly influenced both by object relations thinking and the interpersonal movement. Those groups formulated their clinical visions in reaction to their classical Freudian and Kleinian predecessors; interpersonalists moderated the ideal of an abstinent, paternal, rule-bound analyst and a drive-driven, pleasure-seeking patient while emphasizing its interactive element (e.g., Ehrenberg, 1992; Hirsch, 2014; Sullivan, 1954; Wolstein, 1959). Rejecting the traditional emphasis on drives (sexual and aggressive) along with ideas about interpretive purity and neutrality, they anticipated the relational emphasis on the two-person nature of analytic interaction (Sullivan, 1954). But where interpersonalists saw two adults in interaction, the relational turn expanded this view to address a multiplicity of early, dissociated self-states in relational trauma.

Object relations theorists and self psychologists informed the relational focus on early failure and needed therapeutic provision. But unlike the interpersonalists, they embraced the idea of regression and the analyst's capacity to repair.

Those coming from the interpersonal tradition reacted strongly—and negatively—to models emphasizing this repair element (Aron, 1991, 1992; Hirsch, 2014; Hoffman, 1991; Mitchell, 1984, 1991; D. B. Stern, 1992).[1] Developmental tilt models, embedded in ideas of parental (analytic) repair, seemed to lock the patient into a position of helpless dependence while encouraging the analyst's superiority and analytic certainty.

Rejecting visions of a paternalistic, potentially shame-inducing (classical) analyst and a benevolent, idealized (Winnicottian) one, relational and feminist writers underscored the analyst's ubiquitous—and flawed—subjectivity. She—like the mother—is a person first and last; her subjecthood is to be celebrated rather than excluded (Bassin, 1997, 1999; Bassin, Honey, & Kaplan, 1994; Benjamin, 1986, 1988, 1995a, 1998; Chodorow, 1978; Dimen, 1991; Dinnerstein, 1976; Fast, 1984; Goldner, 1991; Harris, 1991, 1997; Layton, 1998).

Perhaps a bit drunk on the excitement of this new psychoanalytic vision, early relationalists threw away the old book of analytic prescriptions and proscriptions (Hoffman, 1998), or at least whole chapters of it. Interpretations were replaced by enactment—a term first coined by Jacobs (1986), a Freudian influenced by self psychology. When unpacked, enactments were mutative, not destructive. Impasse didn't end analytic process; when mutually explored, it opened it.

Turning classical Freudian and Kleinian theories on their respective heads, we entered the clinical moment with an eye toward our participation in it. Vivid case examples illustrated how early, entrenched relational patterns could be shifted in the here and now. Our ability to probe the intersection between our own and our patient's unconscious experience became the therapeutic linchpin of relational theory. This was a new kind of analytic heroine—one who could save the day by virtue of her emotional accessibility.

The relational movement resulted in a sea change for some of us (including me). It invited us to revisit ideas such as countertransference and consider the clinical potential embedded in what was originally viewed as a therapeutic interference. Here, I want to examine the relational ideal from the inside out; that is, to engage in self-critique with the aim of expanding our understanding of the limits of relational engagement.

---

1  Critiques of the maternal analytic ideal have softened with time (Chapter 2).

## Our relational heroine

Our relational heroine embodies nearly everything that other analytic theories rejected or disavowed. She's so different that she's really an anti-hero: she borrows old tropes, but then disrupts, rewrites, and reverses them (sometimes with an ahistorical sense of radical newness). In a sense, the relational heroine is an *analytic noir* ideal, valorized for the very attributes that once represented flaws: Her subjectivity, even her reactivity, make her a better analyst rather than one needing more analysis.

Like the interpersonalists before her, the relational analyst is real—open, responsive, non-defensive, willing to self-disclose and use those disclosures to deepen the work. But with inspiration came the potential for excess. And we were as guilty of this kind of excess as was/is every other psychoanalytic movement. Rebelling against, rejecting the therapeutic strictures of early analytic times, we idealized much that prior models had sought to control.

Where classical analysts had been enslaved to abstinence, now we were free to be ourselves. Where once we concealed ourselves as much as possible, now we wanted to reveal; memoirs and essays describing the therapeutic impact of self-disclosure proliferated. We focused on the clinical potential inherent in the mutual exploration of reenactments. We rejected, or forgot, the cautionary wisdom about self-disclosure that our forebears had sounded so loudly. We pathologized patients who evaded or resisted our focus on our subjectivity and the reenactments between us.

In delineating our differences with Freudian, interpersonal, and object relations theories, some of us overlooked areas of convergence (for example, Sullivan's (1954) participant observation, Fiscalini's (1994) concept of analytic co-participation, and Kohut's (1971, 1984) selfobject function). We didn't always recognize those Freudian ancestors—including Jacobs (1986), Loewald (1960), and Sandler (1976)—whose work humanized the analytic relationship and explored transference-countertransference dynamics (Mitchell, 2000). Relationalists who critiqued the object relational notion of regression to dependence overlooked Winnicott's (1971) complex vision of the progression away from regression (object relating) toward object usage and Balint's (1968) discussion of malignant regression—of the risks inherent in regression. Some of us stereotyped therapeutic regression as a simple corrective emotional experience and the selfobject function as a simple avoidance of patients' aggression.

I was among those who identified with aspects of object relations theory as we confronted the relational critique (see also Benjamin, 1988; Bromberg, 1979, 1991; Davies, 1994; Ghent, 1992). And I wondered: Were we idealizing explicit intersubjective exchange? Could we make room for patients' need for holding when it collided with that ideal? And could we embrace relational theory while also defining its limits?

## Developmental relationality in 2023

By the mid-1990s, the place of developmental tilt thinking became the subject of active debate among relational writers (Chapter 2). A more nuanced portrait of patient and analyst took shape; it included ideas about nonlinear movement and shifting self-states (Aron, 2001; Benjamin, 2009, 2010; Cooper, 2014; Davies, 2004; Grand, 2000, 2010; Harris, 2005, 2009; Mitchell, 2000; S. A. Pizer, 1998; Seligman, 2003; Stein, 1999; D. B. Stern, 2009). We moved beyond the early stereotype of relational work as located in loud impasse and explicit self-disclosure and of analytic containment as simply gaslighting.

Bromberg's (2011) and Schore's (2011) work on relational co-shaping underscores a similar therapeutic element: The analyst's attention to her own and her patient's process coalesces into a kind of procedural moderating response to the patient's emotional vulnerability and attachment needs. Like holding and "e" enactments (Bass, 2003), relational co-shaping is a continuous background element. It's informed by unconscious (procedural) factors—by continuous, subtle adjustments between analyst and patient that occur in the present moment (D. N. Stern, 2004). Like the Boston Process Change Study Group's (e.g., 1998) "something more," they help ease emotional reactivity and shift implicit relational knowing.

Analytic holding contributes to relational shaping and vice versa: Our procedural—sometimes unconscious—responses inform our conscious efforts to hold. Both operate behind the scenes during active exploratory work, while in moments of more acute distress, they dominate.

## Enactments in a developmental context:
## The relational baby

Probably because early relational writing rejected developmental tilt models, it tended to obfuscate the ways in which relational theory itself is lodged in an implicit model of therapeutic repair organized around the reparative power of the enacted moment.

Enactments, when worked through, represent a kind of relational do-over. We blunder and become the bad object (Davies, 2004). But we're really everything the bad parent was *not* because we're willing to say the unsayable—we're willing to change. In so doing we offer a powerful antidote to the relational configuration(s) that traumatized; what was dissociated reemerges in therapeutic space, where it can be encompassed and metabolized.

Contemporary perspectives on dissociation and shifting self-states (e.g., Bromberg, 2006; D. B. Stern, 2009; Grand, 2000, 2010) support that idea. Even when our patient feels like an adult, she has the capacity—perhaps disavowed, perhaps not—to access and temporarily move into an early self-state. So, while at times we can speak to our patient about her more vulnerable self-states, at other times we need to speak directly to that baby because it's really she who's in the room.

Both holding and relational shaping, themselves corrective emotional experiences, are lodged in the realm of the intersubjective. They're less authoritarian; they coalesce in interaction with the patient rather than originating in an authoritative, diagnostic stance. Still, embodied therein is a reparative ideal that has resonance precisely because of the early experiences it reverses. This is a long way from a simple vision of patient-as-baby or as-adult. What still needs exploration is our understanding of a patient's needs and their sources.

When our patient needs holding, we view her as if in a baby or child self-state. When she's engaged intersubjectively, she's an adult. It's always the baby (in the adult) whom we try to repair. Despite some discussions of the needs of adult patients outside the baby metaphor (Boulanger, 2007; Slochower, 1993, 2011a), we haven't developed an overarching view of acute need as it makes itself known in adulthood. We've largely ignored models (e.g., Erikson, 1950; Kohut, 1984) that extend the developmental arc or address the adult's need for repair (but see Seligman & Shanok, 1996); we haven't fully filled in the gap between baby and adult or integrated the evolution of attachment needs as they're expressed across the lifespan. This remains a project worth undertaking.

### Aloneness in relational space: Pathologized or honored?

Early analytic models lodged in the ideal of neutrality demanded enormous containment on the analyst's part. Constrained from using our subjectivity in the work, we were left to silently contend with it. Sharing our experience reflected countertransference acting out and sent us back to analysis, or at least for consultation. The relational turn provided a creative solution to this problem. Using our subjectivity and mutually exploring enactments didn't shut down analytic process; it deepened and opened it.

But there's always an underbelly. Relational thinking tends to assume that, despite their anxieties and resistances, patients can tolerate, and ultimately will welcome, expressions of our subjectivity. Even if they don't begin treatment with this capacity, with our help they'll get there.

In many ways, I stand behind this vision and its developmental underpinnings. Aiming to help my patient deepen her capacity for intersubjective recognition is a focus that works for me. But like all models, it has its own potentially problematic implications: It runs the risk of ignoring the importance of alone, interior experience within therapeutic space *and* the potentially disruptive impact of mutual engagement. Because while the analysis of enactments is sometimes where it's at, it's also sometimes not (Chapter 1). At times, our patients (and we) want—or need—to be "alone" with someone who mostly stays out (Corbett, 2014; Ogden, 1997; Slochower, 1993, 1994, 1996a, 1996b, 1999, 2004, 2006c, 2013c).

The capacity to be alone and sustain one's interiority is a prerequisite for intersubjective engagement. Yet we tend to locate this need in an early developmental process. We've privileged, indeed idealized, mutuality, and problematized (even negated) what's not intersubjective. This shift has generated a new vision of pathology that pathologizes the wish—or need—for privacy, solitude, for noninteractive analytic experience, as if it's inherently less "mature," less "developed" than intersubjective engagement. I think it's not. Both explicitly intersubjective and private experiences manifest across the lifespan, and both can represent nonpathological ways of being.

## False dichotomies, false caricatures

Like every psychoanalytic theory, relational theory has been the object of caricature. We've been depicted as clinically impulsive, self-referential, superficial, and foreclosing or sidestepping reflective space. These are caricatures rather than accurate descriptions of relational work. But in the absence of clinical thoughtfulness, they're the doors we're prone to walking through.

I think we've persuasively demonstrated that exploring the reenacted element opens therapeutic process. By embracing what's shared and avoiding authoritarian interpretations, the analytic dyad co-sculpts a historical narrative with considerable emotional power and deepens our patient's experience of self and other. But we also risk occluding its problematic edge and foreclosing what doesn't fit. Our investment in demonstrating the clinical power of the present moment and our participation in it can create its own blind spot(s).

Might we be, at moments, too anxious to relinquish our authority and relocate it within the relational matrix? Might we overlook our patient's need for *us* to know, to comfortably hold our authority? Do we fail to examine her mixed feelings about mutual exploration?

Patients sometimes express gratitude when we introduce our experience into analytic dialogue. Still, I wonder whether there's sometimes more to these moments than meets the eye. Might some patients comply with what they perceive to be *our* wish that these moments be helpful? When they say "I'm so glad you told me how you feel," and sidestep their sense of disturbance about that self-disclosure or about our uncertain, mutual stance? Might they sometimes long for us to be more certain, more knowing, more authoritative than our theory seems to allow? And might we be a bit blind to this side of things because it collides with our professional ideal?

No theory is immune to this kind of clinical blindness, though its particulars will vary. Classical analysts may interpret a patient's denial as unconscious confirmation of the accuracy of their interpretation and sidestep the possibility that they're just plain wrong. Relationalists are probably more vulnerable to the opposite risk—to taking too much at face value a patient's affirmation of what we say, or too quickly accepting their criticism of us. There's a possibility that we'll minimize the conflicted dynamics that underlie her apparently fulsome affirmation or rejection of us, our theory, or our way of working.

A further complication: Some patient may need to please us by "getting with" our clinical agenda, whatever its particulars. How this looks will depend on our theory. Patients in a classical or Kleinian analysis may too easily accept interpretations or appear to appreciate a no in response to a request. Patients in a relational analysis are probably far freer to argue with us. But might they not sometimes feel pressure to affirm the value of intersubjective exchange, to please us by engaging with us when really they'd rather not?

It can be tempting to turn a blind eye to this kind of dynamic because of the pleasure it affords us to be idealized (in whatever way we value), to see our theory confirmed. Can we parse our evaluation of the treatment's effectiveness from our pleasurable response to our patient's appreciation?

Analytic self-interest is implicated here. Whatever our theory, our investment in having the treatment go the way we believe it should can render us a bit deaf. We want something (whether self-affirmation, confirmation that we're "correct," closeness, authentic engagement, or a here-and-now interaction) and so we want our patient to want it too. We look for evidence that she does; we're tempted to accept things at face value when they fit our theory and/or our personal idiom. Will we become inattentive to the ways in which it derails or obfuscates?

## Relational ideals and the idealized dyad

Although caricatures are often veiled attacks, it's also possible to caricature in the opposite direction by exaggerating the positive and ignoring what's not. In addition to ignoring our (and our patient's) wish and need for privacy and solitude, relational theory idealizes the analyst's relational capacity.

The relational ideal envisions an analyst with considerable emotional depth, resilience, and self-reflectivity. She's both eager and able to examine herself and her process; when she hits a roadblock, she aims to openly reflect on it and then move past it. This is an ideal worth embracing. It invites us to examine our impact and consider the possibility that we're responsible for the current therapeutic roadblock. Yet it's not without an underbelly.

Our ideal collides with an inconvenient clinical truth—that it's not only our patient who isn't always up for, open to, or capable of deep emotional engagement *or* of reflectively considering why we're not. That we're not consistently able to recognize our flaws and defenses. Despite our commitment to dyadic engagement and despite the satisfaction we derive from the intimacy it allows, there are times when the shared analysis of enactments is the last thing we want. At times, our need for self-protection and privacy surfaces and forecloses our wish or need for mutual exchange (Grand, 2010). This professional ideal can exaggerate our intersubjective capacity and minimize the obstacles that stand between us (analyst and patient) and ongoing relational engagement.

Inevitably, our analytic ideal will sometimes collide with our wish—and need—to change, to make contact, to do something useful. Those collisions emerge, independent of our theoretical allegiance, out of the space between the professional ideal to which we aspire and the reality of our human fallibility.

Every theoretical model idealizes something. Relational theory idealizes intersubjectivity and excludes its problematic edge; classical models idealize interpretive neutrality and can miss the element of withholding or penetrating attack it embodies. Self psychology and holding models are vulnerable to sidestepping the negative transference-countertransference. You get the idea.

At its best, the relational ideal includes a recognition that it's elusive: Even if we aim for ongoing mutual exploration, we know we can't ever entirely get there. Full disclosure is impossible because we analysts have our own unconscious—and unformulated—experience. It's also undesirable; no matter how much we value intersubjectivity, there will always be information, feelings, experiences that we choose not to share because of our wish for privacy and/or because we suspect it would be too disturbing or hurtful to do otherwise. We choose (partially unconsciously) how we engage and how we contain based on a mixture of our patient's and our own needs, wishes, and anxieties, along with our clinical ideas about what's therapeutic and what's not. It's when we lose track of these complexities that we slide toward excess. Can we balance the ideal of analytic openness against our personal limits *and* against the value of privacy? Certainly, relational theory is so thoroughly grounded in the value of exploring our failings that we ought to be better at this than those who embrace a differently idealized analytic vision. And often we are. But not always.

In our enthusiastic embrace of what was previously forbidden, we haven't always paid sufficient attention to the less-than-obvious impact of freely speaking politics, sex, hate, love; in fact, of our freely speaking. We didn't always consider the potentially disturbing impact of analytic self-disclosure. Or of teaching new candidates the value of waiting and listening until they've gotten the lay of the emotional landscape, or of carefully investigating underlying dynamics before playfully introducing what might be disruptive.

No, I'm not suggesting we return to a traditional treatment model; we'd lose far more than we'd gain. First, analytic restraint too often coalesces into a kind of holding back that itself embodies a sado-masochistic enactment. Second, even if we think restraint is desirable, it's not always achievable. There are moments when our countertransference erupts—for better and for worse. To further complicate things, restraint is no therapeutic panacea: Like analytic silence, restraint can be gaslighting, mystifying, can demand compliance or trigger dissociation. There's no evading our impact, whether enacted or implicit.

But these caveats also may obfuscate the fact that analysts can do real harm by doing. Csillag (2014) illustrates this: She became traumatically derailed by her analyst's engagement in political arguments while he remained unaware of the toxic effect it was having. His belief in openness made him blind to its excesses, to the possibility that staying out would have been a wiser analytic stance.

Just last week, my new patient John described something similar: His therapist expressed an envious and competitive reaction to John's recent professional success, indicating that he felt it would have been dishonest *not* to self-disclose. Although John felt disturbed and unsafe, he expressed appreciation for the analyst's honesty and didn't articulate his upset reaction to the disclosure.

But now feeling constrained and silenced, John soon quit therapy, offering an excuse (a demanding new job) his therapist accepted at face value. Because the analyst's self-disclosure fit his theory of therapeutic action, he didn't consider the possibility that something more lay beneath what had seemed so intimate and helpful. A clinical blind spot with theoretical origins.

Allowing ourselves to examine our patient's dynamics outside the realm of the intersubjective offers us an additional point of clinical entrée that can coexist with an ongoing study of the co-created element. As Nancy McWilliams (e.g., 2011, 2017) lucidly illustrates, it's possible to think about diagnosis psychoanalytically *and* include the intersubjective in our thinking. By addressing individual character style in interface and collision with our relational perspective, we deepen and complicate our clinical point of entrée. Because relationalists can both engage *and* stay out. We're capable of refraining from saying the unsayable, jointly exploring our countertransference or breaking into our patient's process or her illusions about us. We can allow for a zone of deniability—an arena that allows her *not* to see what cannot be metabolized. It's here that analytic restraint opens therapeutic space, rather than constricting it, by making room for that need.

Of course, our move toward restraint isn't uniquely informed by our understanding of the patient; it's also shaped by our own need not to know, be known, or to challenge. In this sense, restraint is as dynamically complex as intersubjectivity.

It's here that the relational ideal of analytic uncertainty—of ongoing self-reflection—can stand us in good stead; it supports self-examination and openness to the ways our clinical choice—whether to express or contain—was influenced by our own dynamics.

I thus want to include the ideal of analytic restraint within the relational umbrella without elevating it to a primary or dominant place. Certainly, most analytic enactments can be worked through and repaired. *But not all.* Some enactments are boundary violations—sexual and nonsexual. They do lasting harm and cannot be usefully analyzed. This is an omnipresent danger for all of us, no matter what our clinical theory. While relationalists are no more vulnerable to committing major boundary violations than those who adhere to a different theory, we're also no less vulnerable. In acknowledging all this, we invite respectful—rather than competitive— intertheoretical dialogue that includes an appreciation of areas of commonality and difference.

It's my hope that writers from other orientations will engage in a similar kind of self-critique, that we'll address the risks associated with *every* position, including our own tendency to move too quickly toward the enacted therapeutic dimension. Because our intertheoretical conversations can be organized *not* in argument with our psychoanalytic Other but with the aim of respectfully delineating our differences while also deepening areas of commonality.

## Postscript

This essay, written about ten years ago, represented a response to what I then viewed as relational theory's clinical overreach. Today (2023), far fewer essays are organized around the unshaded value of self-disclosure *or* against restraint. Things have softened, and while I don't think we can take for granted the arguments I made, I also see far less "excess" today than I did when I wrote it. We're far more able to encompass both positions without resorting to the polarization of earlier times.

# Chapter 5

# A few regrets

Psychoanalytic critique is nearly always organized around what's wrong with the *other* theory. That other theory is too . . . focused on aggression, on sex, on the countertransference, on self-experience. *Those* analysts make too few—or too many—interpretations. Their model is rigid, self-indulgent, narrow. Our own theory has it right.

This isn't a difficulty unique to any specific theory; it's endemic to the field. Indeed, since our psychoanalytic beginnings, our models have been formulated in conversation (often in argument) with their theoretical predecessors and competitors. We sculpt a vision of the kind of analyst we want to be and the kind of change we hope to effect; there's an implicit (if not overt) rebuke aimed at the other theory—and analyst—buried (or not so buried) within that vision. Psychoanalytic factionalism dominates (Chapter 12).

Theoretical comparisons aren't intrinsically bad. They have the potential to deepen our thinking and sharpen our engagement with a range of issues (Aron, 2017). But despite the generative element embedded in cross-theoretical critique, these comparisons also have a downside. To elevate the originality of our own contribution, we exaggerate difference and rigidify the core principles to which we adhere. We minimize, sometimes denigrate, the position of the psychoanalytic Other whose ideals collide—or overlap excessively—with our own. Why have so many theories emerged in counterpoint to—if not in rebellion against—their predecessors? Is the "anxiety of influence" (Bloom, 1973) intrinsic to theory building?

I want to move past the intertheoretical battles of earlier days and toward critical *self*-examination. I use the word "critical" here in what I view as its best sense; a thoughtful, non-defensive examination of the limitations and excesses of one's own position. Self-critique can deepen

DOI: 10.4324/9781032691534-7

our understanding of our theory and its overlaps with alternative models. Here I consider the limitations and problematic edges of my own theory of relational holding.

It's not surprising that Winnicott didn't explore how the analyst's subjectivity impacts the clinical moment. Winnicott wrote in pre-relational times; analytic asymmetry was a theoretical given. Despite his (1947, 1949, 1955) acknowledgment of maternal and analytic hate and the strain they place on the analyst, Winnicott believed that the analyst could assess when—and how—to hold. Left to be explored was holding's dyadic element—the ways in which the analytic couple together establishes and sustains a holding experience. Also missing was an exploration of how our subjectivity informs our moves in and out of holding.

The relational holding model described in chapters 1 and 2 bridges the apparent collision between Winnicottian and early relational thinking. It also embeds a relational aim: Holding strengthens processes of self-reflectivity, affect elaboration, and regulation; all capacities that underlie our tolerance for, and enjoyment of, free engagement with the other (i.e., a capacity for object usage). Over time, holding will open the way to analytic mutuality. Further, holding and intersubjective work aren't dichotomous; these threads alternate rapidly and fluidly. And patients sometimes feel held *by* an interpretation (Winnicott, 1986).

The move toward or away from holding isn't purely diagnostic. It implicates the analyst because her clinical choice is informed by her need not to know, be known, or to challenge. The element of restraint intrinsic to holding, then, is as dynamically informed as intersubjective exchange. It's here that the relational ideal of analytic uncertainty—of ongoing self-reflectivity—stands us in good stead; it reminds us that every clinical choice—whether to express or contain—is influenced both by dyadic enactments and our own dynamics.

## Revisiting the holding-expressivity binary

While the concept of relational holding added to the relational perspective, I've come to believe that it also furthered—or at least retained—some problematic elements. Like theories that came before (and like those that will come after), it represented an overcorrection to previous excesses. I think it's time for another correction, one that provides an additional element of theoretical/clinical balance.

First, the theoretical. On one level, holding and mutuality exist in tension with each other. After all, we can't both tell *and* not tell our patient how we're experiencing her in the clinical moment. We can't both bracket *and* express our subjectivity.

Or can we? When we articulate our "separate" understanding of a patient, we attend to the therapeutic impact of directly using our subjectivity and dynamic understanding. When we hold, we focus on the therapeutic impact of containment. In both instances, we emphasize those aspects of our work (holding or expressivity) that align with our preferred theory. We also skip over—or at least minimize—the therapeutic potential of the other clinical dimension.

I want to further deconstruct the holding-expressivity binary: Because, despite our best attempts at containment, aspects of our personhood seep into the therapeutic arena no matter how good we are at working within a holding frame. In this sense, our capacity to hold is always partial; our patient picks up on our subjectivity even when we're doing our best to bracket it. Further, we inadvertently disclose—and fail to disclose—things about ourselves and/or our feelings *despite* a different conscious intention. And the same is true of relational exchange: Even as we bring ourselves into the clinical moment, there are things we refrain from expressing (perhaps deliberately; perhaps procedurally).

I'm suggesting that holding and explicit intersubjective exchange each embodies considerable expressivity *and* considerable restraint. These joint processes coexist as figure and ground in every treatment. Each shifts imperceptibly as analyst and patient react and adjust to the other.

## What leaks when we hold?

Sonia phoned me weeping, very unusual for her. It was a Sunday, and she'd had a huge fight with her partner and was enormously distressed. After empathizing with her upset, I softly added that her hurt reflected both anger and terror about being abandoned—feelings that were emerging as central themes in our work. Sonia responded with recognition and relief; she felt held because I resonated with her upset *and* because I named its sources in a way Sonia could recognize but hadn't yet identified. In this sense, there was a holding element embedded both in my empathy and in my interpretation.

Now Sonia began to speak about an early experience of abandonment that she connected with her current distress. But here my subjectivity collided with Sonia's; I didn't want to prolong our conversation, I wanted to get back to my Sunday. As gently as I could, I interrupted her, saying I needed to get off the phone; I knew she wasn't ready to say goodbye, but we'd talk more on Tuesday.

On Tuesday we returned to the phone call. Sonia said that she appreciated my understanding but was upset that I got off the phone so quickly. She added, half teasingly, that she guessed I had a life too and she wasn't sure she liked that. We laughed, but we both knew that something quite serious was being opened. For the first time, Sonia named her awareness of my subjectivity and was able to tolerate my separateness, albeit unhappily. This didn't mean (to me) that Sonia no longer needed holding, but rather that she was beginning to shift toward a more complex (intersubjective) view of me and of our relationship.

Of course, I'm describing the manifest (conscious) dimension of this clinical moment; less clear are the underlying enacted or unconscious dynamics that informed it. Might my holding response have emerged out of a wish to remain in an idealized position? Or—and—did my wish to end the call reflect my discomfort with the parental role I felt pulled into? Was I unconsciously put off by Sonia's intense neediness? And what about Sonia? Did we enact something of her own longing *and* discomfort with an early wish by quickly ending the conversation? That is, had I temporarily "become" both the soothing *and* rejecting parent of Sonia's childhood?

### What we hold when we express

Just as aspects of our personhood seep into the holding space despite our efforts to bracket what's disjunctive, nondisclosure or restraint may turn up despite our commitment to intersubjective engagement.

Steven spent a session describing his critical feelings about his supervisor, someone I knew and liked (this isn't something Steven could have known). Although I ordinarily worked with Steven outside the holding metaphor (i.e., I felt free to interpret, confront, and articulate my thoughts and reactions to what he said), I found myself trying to bracket my somewhat defensive reaction to Steven's view of my colleague. I was aware that Steven might have picked this up but chose not to tell Steven about our relationship, partly to make space for his own feelings, partly to protect my privacy, and partly out of my own defensiveness. Here, then, was an instance in which my subjectivity shifted my clinical stance away from the interactive exploration I ordinarily did with Steven[1].

More than before, I'm convinced every clinical moment embodies an element of analytic expressivity *and* an element of holding, though only one predominates. We can never say *everything* (in or out of the consulting room); even when we self-disclose or address an enactment, we choose (unconsciously or deliberately) not to disclose something else. We may bracket what we sense would be too hurtful or disruptive to our patient. (In part, that's why I didn't disclose to Steven my relationship with his supervisor). But we also bracket for our own reasons—because *we* would feel embarrassed, ashamed, or endangered were we to acknowledge our subjectivity.

No matter how committed we are to a holding model, then, we sometimes disclose (advertently, inadvertently, unconsciously, or not). And no matter how committed we are to mutuality we don't tell our patients everything all the time. We choose (both implicitly and deliberately) what to say—and when. And what not to say. So, we hold even when we disclose. And disclose even when we hold. I think this is true for those who believe in radical analytic openness *and* for those committed to a holding model. And those in between, of course.

Another complication that needs unpacking: Our patient rarely experiences our shifts toward and away from holding in as predictable a way as our theory (and wish) might suggest. She may, for example, feel held when we actively enter the clinical conversation. She may feel directly engaged when we're trying to hold. It's this doubleness—*holding and analytic expressivity*—that accounts for the multiplicity of self and mutual experience.

While many of us embrace this doubleness on a theoretical level, we tend to teach our candidates in ways that retain and even rigidify the holding-expressivity binary. Those who tilt toward holding or containment are unlikely to theorize the clinical impact of the expressivity it embodies. Those who emphasize mutuality tend not to theorize the clinical power of the background holding they're simultaneously doing. We focus on the

---

1 It's equally true that explicit relational engagement can emerge out of the analyst's desire to know and be known.

impact of our preferred theory and miss, overlook, or avoid fully examining its underbelly. In so doing, we further the binary and implicitly ask our candidates to take sides. Both sides miss something.

It's been extraordinarily difficult for our training institutes to do both—to teach candidates a particular (preferred) theory while simultaneously addressing that theory's limitations. For relational Winnicottians like me, this means training candidates to be on the lookout for the potentially gaslighting effect of holding—the ways we signal that our patient shouldn't see what she sees about us. For those who emphasize the therapeutic impact of mutuality, it means training them to watch out for evidence of disturbed, disavowed reactions to our expressivity. And since we all work, to some extent, in both ways, we need to teach candidates to do both; that is, to find the holding element embedded in mutuality and the expressivity embedded in holding.

## Analytic babies and adults: Beyond another binary

By emphasizing vulnerable patients' need for holding, I left another old but problematic clinical assumption partly unpacked; namely, that the patient is either a relatively sturdy adult who can tolerate explicit intersubjective/mutual exchange *or* a baby needing holding. To some extent, this clinical tilt persists even though we've largely rejected unidimensional visions of patient-as-baby and recognize the presence of baby states in the adult patient (Chapter 2).

In the consulting room we tend to move toward and away from the "need" element depending on whether we experience our patient as in an adult or in a baby self-state; or/and depending on whether our patient seems to be inviting us to enter the analytic dialogue as parent, peer, or child. Those working within a holding frame may miss the defensive function of a baby self-state that covers over a more grown-up and conflicted one. Those who privilege intersubjective engagement may miss the baby state lurking behind an apparently adult self-presentation that masks a self-protective layer.

We're all vulnerable to ignoring the limitations of our clinical vision, whatever its particulars. It's difficult to decenter—to remain alert to the multiple clinical threads present in the room. Certainly, at any moment, only one is foregrounded. But the others are rarely absent; they lurk in the background and are easy to miss. This binary (patient as baby or adult)—a consequence of another iteration of the clinical/theoretical pendulum swing—probably couldn't have been deconstructed until it was well established. But in the clearer light of hindsight, I want to unpack and complicate it.

## Holding and the idealized analyst

There's a related problem embedded in most clinical theories, including my ideas about relational holding. It's an unarticulated idealization of the analyst's emotional capacity and ability to know what to do—and when. We assume we can respond to intense affect states with the necessary containment. To meet our patient where she is. This analytic ideal is organized around an elevated vision of our capacity for empathic attunement. It privileges the mutative effect of relational repair: Our patient gets better in the context of who we are, what we do and don't do. I remain convinced of the therapeutic potential in this kind of process. But.

Independent of our theory, we risk inflating our reparative power and sidestepping the possibility that we won't be able to provide enough holding (or, from a different perspective, enough relational engagement, sufficiently penetrating interpretations, etc.) to sustain things. That the work may become too much—too burdensome, anxiety-producing, or frustrating. There's a risk we'll respond to the pressure we're feeling by rebelling, "acting out," by inserting ourselves in ways that cannot be encompassed when we're trying to hold, or by withdrawing when we're trying to engage. Of using interpretations in a retaliatory way or deflecting our own (or our patient's) anger by determinedly remaining in an idealized position.

Analytic idealizations take multiple shapes. Holding models idealize the analyst's capacity for containment. Interactive clinical models idealize the analyst's capacity to be self-reflective and open. Classical models idealize the analyst's interpretive wisdom and nonreactivity. Kleinian models idealize the analyst's ability to use her countertransference interpretively. Self psychology, the analyst's capacity to fully enter the patient's experience. Stepping back from our preferred theory requires that we engage and challenge the particular idealizations we've unthinkingly embraced.

## Another look at regression and its underbelly

I was in analytic training in the early 1980s when my object relational and Freudian supervisors introduced me to Winnicott's concept of regression to dependence. The patient's need to access and dwell in early states was a clinical given, to be allowed, sometimes invited. I wasn't taught to worry about it.

I started worrying later. Today I see regression as both powerful *and* problematic. On one hand, analytic process can create a space within which early, disavowed, or dissociated trauma states are contacted and a new beginning (Balint, 1968) takes shape. Over the years, I've lived through this kind of process with people whose lives were transformed as a result.

But significant risk can accompany it. A regressed patient has something (sometimes a lot) to lose in the present. No matter how well I hold. Her sense of intactness may be threatened; her capacity to sustain contact with adult self-experience may attenuate or even disappear. My centrality in her emotional life may interfere with her investment in other relationships. And when prolonged, regression can put relationships, jobs, and ordinary functioning on the line.

I'm *not* referring to what Balint called a malignant regression. I'm talking about the clinical risk embedded in a needed therapeutic regression of whatever affective shape. Because holding locates the analyst at the center of the patient's emotional life in ways that we don't (that I didn't) always query: The analyst who holds (in whatever way she does) privileges her patient's reliance on the analyst's capacity to contain over a focus on her patient's emotional autonomy. Even when my patient moves through and beyond her reliance on my holding function, there's something else that may not be addressed: namely, difficulty with self-regulation.

My supervisee Andrea has been working with Mona for about a year. Mona was overready for a regression; her previous analyst had died suddenly, just when Mona was becoming dependent on her. Shortly after beginning treatment with Andrea, Mona recovered memories of her mother's early abandonment and became flooded by the symbolic repetition embedded in her analyst's death. She expressed intense baby longings toward Andrea and asked for daily sessions.

On one hand, this rich and deep work helped Mona identify, organize, and master the early trauma. But Mona's reliance on Andrea came at a price; any interruption in their schedule left her acutely dysregulated. Mona's shame about her baby longings also left her unable to turn to friends or family for support. Mona was similarly unwilling to use medication or other adjunctive therapy to manage things and responded to Andrea's suggestions as rejection ("You don't want the responsibility anymore"). The regression deepened; Mona was barely functioning. Alarmed, Andrea and I worried that Mona would lose her job and was putting her good-enough relationship at risk. Happily, though, Mona came out of the regression before things fell apart. As she restabilized, Andrea said, "I think we dodged a bullet. Should I—could I—have known? Should I have tried to stop the regression? Will there be a price to pay down the road?"

*Had* Andrea missed something important when she allowed (invited) Mona to rely so heavily on her holding capacity? Had Mona and Andrea unconsciously evaded examining Mona's conflicted attachment or other dynamic issues? Had Mona's investment in remaining a "good object" muddied things?

Because of our investment in working the way we do, we run the risk of unconsciously prolonging a holding experience because it feels good to *us*. Or of failing to address—directly and/or interpretively—conflicted aspects of a patient's attachment. We may not recognize the defensive element embedded in her emotional helplessness.

When we hold, we try to provide and/or support a regulating function, while (at least temporarily) setting aside work around a patient's self-regulatory capacity. And while—ideally—the holding process will become internalized and integrated, this doesn't always happen. Like analysis interminable (Freud, 1937), we run the risk of allowing our patient's dependence to block engagement in the world for too long, of remaining within a protected clinical space that excludes too much. Will the fantasy that our sensitivity and holding capacity are all our patient needs obscure holding's underbelly the way it can occlude patients' need to develop and sustain agency?

Of course, we can hold and keep an eye on all this. We can explore the defensive use of dependence. We can address patients' fear of separating and/or of losing us even as we hold. And we can work on affect regulation even as we hold.

I'm increasingly aware of how essential the latter work is; I attend more than before to the development of a capacity for self-holding alongside patients' need to access and articulate "being" self-states. By self-holding, I don't refer to Winnicott's (1960a) emphasis on its defensive function. Certainly, we analysts need to engage in self-holding (really, in self-regulation). Further, self-holding *can* reflect an overactive false self in Winnicott's sense. But some patients need help developing their own capacities for affect regulation and emotional resilience (Grand, 2017b) even as we try to provide a holding space. Were I to rewrite my own work, I'd integrate a focus on issues of "doing," affect regulation, and resilience alongside holding.

Whatever our preferred clinical model, our own needs and dynamics inform the position we take and can obscure others. Thus, for example, a belief in the value of holding may reflect our need for a certain kind of relationship. It can camouflage the ways that holding leaves a patient feeling abandoned or "un-held." It can make us blind to the ways she needs to feel more of *us*, of our subjectivity, or more of our capacity to draw a clinical line. This is holding's underbelly.

## Holding in changing analytic times

There's been a broad shift in the psychoanalytic zeitgeist, at least in the eastern United States, away from daily sessions and toward twice, or at most, three times weekly treatment. Most people don't want or cannot manage—practically and/or financially—to come more often. This shift amplifies the risks associated with a regression to dependence. In the absence of frequent sessions, an intense relationship with the analyst is harder to contain within the treatment space. It's more likely to leak. And not every life, family, or career can contain a partial, much less a full, regression to dependence.

All this, pre-Covid. Today, many of us work outside the realm of embodied experience; the protected therapeutic space we were accustomed to is no more. Remote work confronts us with a range of impingements on therapeutic process including—but not limited to—internet instability that breaks up our voice, image, or both; children and animals that barge into the "treatment room." Not to mention the sociopolitical crises that regularly invade therapeutic space. All this can disrupt the kind of holding experience some patients need (Chapter 11).

Whether we'll adapt to the virtual despite the absent (or at least distorted) mirror neuron function (cf. Schore, 2003a, 2003b) remains to be seen. Some feel frustrated and limited by a screen-based relationship. But others experience it differently. A colleague recently told me about a highly defended patient who started having his daily (Zoom) sessions from his bed; he's become regressed in a way that's clinically useful. Teletherapy has opened the door to a deeper treatment experience for him.

To return to the broader question: Even when (if) we return to our offices, can we create the same kind of protected holding space we took for granted in earlier analytic times? Will the shift toward flexible working hours and the option of working from home—both brought about by Covid—carry forward and make more space for intensive treatment? Or will life's intensified pressure block the luxury of a regression to dependence?

In part, my increased caution about therapeutic regression emerges from contemporary interpersonal and relational thinking in tandem with the sociocultural shift emphasizing autonomy. We've moved away from a simple self-identification as reparative parental object and toward a more complex view of patient-as-adult. My emphasis on helping people develop a sense of agency may also reflect the contemporary neoliberal position idealizing individual autonomy and self-regulation. Aron (personal communication, 2016) believed that this focus on autonomy emerged in the early post-World War II era when both returning GIs and Holocaust refugees were forced to manage under horrifying circumstances. They had no choice but to adapt to a new world alone—a challenge requiring agency and autonomy that left little room for dependence.

Personal and clinical experience are also implicated in my shift away from holding a regression. Here's how: The hopeful enthusiasm with which I entered this field has been tempered by time. In part, experience has shown me how much change psychoanalysis can effect and how powerful the holding process can be. But along with that awareness came others that were less affirming. While some people made deep and rapid use of analytic process and particularly of holding experiences, others got stuck, didn't change much, and/or were acutely dependent on my holding function over (what seemed to me) too long a time. Their capacity to self-regulate remained limited. On the other hand, and to my surprise, some people who came only once a week changed as much as—sometimes more than—did those in four-times-weekly analysis. I began to question the therapeutic necessity of intense treatment frequency and became more aware of its problematic potential. I wanted to help patients do some of the work on their own and find ways to manage emotional disruption between sessions. All this moved me a bit away from a focus on the holding element.

And then there was me. As a young analyst, I tried hard to meet my patients where they were. When I was 39, I arranged for a suicidal patient to phone me daily while I was out of the country on vacation. She relied on the ongoing calls, stayed out of the hospital, and ultimately got better (I describe my work with Sarah in Slochower, 1992, 1996c, 2014d). The contact seemed essential given Sarah's suicidality; indeed, it never really occurred to me to do otherwise. A few years later, another patient—not so much regressed as massively anxious and urgent—managed time between our three weekly sessions by leaving me long phone messages on my pre-digital answering machine. She often ran out my tape. I didn't mind much; I was aware of her desperation and need for containment. And she, too, got better.

Today I'd mind doing both. I'm far more cognizant of my own clinical/personal limits and more aware of the problematic edge to a kind of responsiveness that once felt simply necessary. Of the risk that my patient will become reliant on my soothing capacity in a way that truncates her own. That I'll participate in a fantasy that has its own dynamic underpinnings for us both.

I also have an intensified awareness of—and need for—time (Chapter 11). Time alone, time with grandchildren and children, to exercise, write, travel. For quiet evenings. When I was in my 30s and 40s, I didn't feel this way and I didn't get it. Indeed, I have a vivid memory of my experience as a patient at that time. I had asked my own analyst for an extra session I felt I needed; she said no and explained that she wanted time for herself—to have a coffee, to relax. I remember feeling more puzzled than upset. What was the big deal about adding a single session to her week? I just didn't understand. I thought she was being rigid (and on one level, she was). But I couldn't think about what was going on between us (and in her) that might have informed that rigidity.

Today, my identification has shifted away from that of patient to analyst—and an older analyst at that. And so, while I can provide a theoretical rationale for the legitimacy of this clinical shift, it's also personally derived. It reflects a different experience of time, an awareness that comes with aging, along with personality and temperament, of course. And with the emergence of different necessities associated with it. With the recognition that I won't be here forever, and neither will my patients; that I need to do what I can to help them change *now*.

After all, I started thinking and writing about the holding theme a long time ago. I was, alas, a whole lot younger then. More taken with the romance embedded in the Winnicottian metaphor. Less focused on the limitations of analytic process or on helping people develop their own sturdiness outside it. And certainly, far less aware that time is of the essence.

I want to underscore that when I speak of regret, I'm not speaking from a place of remorse, loss, or guilt. Or sadness. To the contrary. I'm talking about looking back *and* forward with a clearer eye. About how time alters, clarifies, and sometimes corrects our earlier understanding of things. Because regret is *not* self-reproach. To have regret, to name and own it, feels central to my psychoanalytic ideal. It's what stands between me and a rigidity that too easily morphs into a kind of calcified, defensive clinical position. It is, in my view, a sort of theoretical capacity for concern in the Winnicottian sense. I rejoice at the opportunity to revisit and revise my own thinking, to identify my clinical/theoretical moments of overreach. To reflect on how time and experience have shaped and reshaped my thinking.

It's in this spirit that I articulate these regrets: I wish I had more fully unpacked and theorized the interpenetration of holding and explicit mutual engagement. I wish I had focused on the move from holding not merely toward intersubjective recognition, but toward self-regulation. Not to minimize holding's clinical power, but to include the vulnerability it doesn't address.

A wish that lies beneath these regrets is that we could all—whatever our theory—engage in self, rather than cross-theoretical, critique. It's a wish for the kind of self-exploratory engagement that doesn't reflect an assumption that we—whoever we are—represent the analytic Second Coming. That we could use self-critique, move beyond splitting and negating the *other* way of working toward genuinely inner *and* intersubjective theoretical dialogue.

# Part 2

# Pushing the Envelope
## How Far Is Too Far?

# Introduction

Andrea Celenza

## Transgressions are us

We tend toward strong opinions when it comes to sexual boundary violations. Convictions, really. A veritable 11th commandment, this conviction encompasses a certainty that arises from within and functions as a signal, a warning, and a firewall—"Thou shalt not do *that*!" In one fell swoop we rid ourselves of the impurities that live in our psyche and find momentary relief, self-satisfaction (if not a sense of superiority) that we are above the day-to-day struggles and transgressions (major and minor) that characterize our work. Would if that were true.

But we are drawn to transgress! We wouldn't need a commandment if this were not the case. Joyce wants to reckon with this push/pull and has written a book that shatters illusions and exposes what we'd rather not see. This exposure is a good thing and not traumatic—our perfectionist illusions weigh us down and foreclose deep thinking. They prevent understanding our humanity. I remember an interaction with my analyst when I thought his attention was flagging. I wanted him to listen carefully to me every second. (I was sitting up at the time so I could monitor him.) He said he could promise 95 percent of his attention every session. I told him that was fine for his other patients, but it was not good enough for me . . . I wanted 100 percent. He replied, "And when I'm with my other patients, attending to them 95 percent of the time, I can think about you in the remaining 5 percent!)" It was funny at the time and all too real. I had to accept his version of imperfection, limits . . . and separateness.

Joyce writes about that symbolic 5 percent (a percentage that is, in reality, much larger). She wants psychoanalytic work to be *real*. She comes by her penchant for truth, integrity, and affective responsivity honestly—her parents were both psychoanalysts with their offices in the family home.

DOI: 10.4324/9781032691534-9

Not only was dinner conversation jargon-filled (in true psychoanalytic fashion), Joyce witnessed *real* psychoanalysts at work—not ideal or perfect, but human. No doubt this was all part of her growth-promoting and de-idealizing reckoning in her journey toward adulthood and that pesky depressive position (sigh).

Joyce refuses idealizations and omnipotence. After all, she grew up that way. Idealization prevents metabolizing the disillusionments with our mentors (some of whom are now violators). This conflicts with the vision of the omnipotent analyst working 80 hours per week. In effect, we cherish our ideals more than we do our self-care. Joyce emphasizes community as part of self-care—made up of trusted others with whom we can reveal our misdemeanors as well as level-headed supervisors who will not react punitively if we share erotic countertransferences. Her emphasis on the need for community (preferably, small groups) is not just any community but one that accepts our various occupational hazards (other-centeredness, self-deprivation, fantasies of rescue, depletion, burnout, and omnipotence) and can hold such clinical hazards as inevitable sequela of inordinate dedication and isolation.

This is especially needed now that our industry is becoming so feminized. . . . We can no longer view the problem of violations (especially sexual) as the work of toxic masculinity or within the sole province of psychopathic predators. The rise in female transgressors is disturbing but should not come as a surprise (Celenza, 2022a).

Joyce has always written from the point of view of the analyst and in this way, she is an analyst's analyst. She is one of the few writers who delves into *our own* psyche, tooling around to see where motives lie, what hides in secret corners, and from where we draw inspiration. She has accepted imperfection and prefers it to idealization, thereby making her writing genuinely helpful. In the following three chapters, she writes about the ways in which the analyst can implicitly and secretly coerce the analysand into collusive exploitative relationships—from ordinary enactments to open or secret misdemeanors (perhaps her most famous paper on this subject) to the most egregious sexual boundary violations.

Joyce adds her voice to the few who write about establishing a restorative justice system, including supportive and reparative processes so that analysts-at-risk *behind* the couch do not become analysts *on* the couch or those who ignore what we'd prefer to exclude. One of the salutary effects of our efforts in this vein inheres in the fact that analysts and therapists are coming forward more frequently for consultation and support when they fear they *might* become sexually involved with a patient. What better outcome could we hope for?

Analyses happen in a highly unusual mode of relating within the context of external reality (not in an insulated bubble). Multiplicity helps in theorizing, but the truth of the matter is a certain kind of messiness. Does a clean break preserve an idealization? Do post-analytic contacts continue it? Is "graduation" to a post-analytic relationship a form of nepotism or an invitation to a new kind of equality or mutuality? What if the analysand wants to return to analysis? I surmise this can be done if a healthy flexibility had been cultivated throughout (see Modell, 1990; Celenza, 2014, 2022b). In this way, Joyce's analytic ideals embody realistic goals, including post-treatment sequels and the underlying flexibility implied where multiple pathways for relating are held as mature capacities.

We all come to this profession with very personal and largely unconscious sensibilities. Perhaps in line with my Italian upbringing, I found a passionate home in psychoanalysis. For Joyce, making a psychoanalytic home was about a fierce confrontation to corrupt authority that was, in true Winnicottian and Sullivanian fashion, at once real and much more human than otherwise.

# Chapter 6

# The analyst's secret delinquencies

Dr. M, a supervisee with whom I've been working for several years, opened our session with a confession she made with some difficulty. Before I describe it, let me contextualize things a bit. Dr. M is a sensitive, skilled analyst who's been in the field for nearly two decades. She seeks out supervision despite considerable expertise, less because she feels clinically insecure than because she believes it enriches her work. We had worked together for five years, and I knew her to be a serious professional with an impeccable sense of commitment to her patients. For all these reasons, I found her confession jarring.

About ten minutes into a telephone session, Dr. M's patient, Mr. J, interrupted himself to ask about "a weird sound" he heard, saying it resembled pages in a magazine being turned. Mr. J's guess was correct; Dr. M was, in fact, quietly skimming through magazines and catalogues and giving Mr. J less than her full attention. On the spot and intensely guilty, Dr. M lied; she said that she was taking notes on the session and had been turning the pages of her notebook. Mr. J seemed to accept her explanation easily and returned to describing other experiences.

Before I address the complex dynamics embedded in this enactment, let me underscore that Dr. M is far from alone in her secret delinquency. Although seldom acknowledged in public forums, Dr. M's action is one of many common infractions of the analytic contract. Yet, despite a burgeoning literature on serious ethical violations, we haven't examined the dynamics underlying less egregious yet still worrisome collisions of professional ethics and self-interest. Probably because analytic misdemeanors seldom disrupt the treatment on a permanent basis *and* because they're nevertheless unacceptable, these acts are infrequently discussed and rarely written about.

DOI: 10.4324/9781032691534-10

By characterizing some therapeutic actions as delinquencies, I'm focusing on those professional behaviors that are secretively—and often guiltily—enacted. I use the term "delinquencies" to refer to moments when we momentarily, but with apparently conscious intent, deliberately disengage from the treatment process to satisfy a personal need. Although some delinquencies occur during face-to-face sessions, it's my impression that most are intentionally hidden, committed either when a patient is on the couch or during phone or virtual sessions. In minor and more egregious ways, we exploit an opportunity to secretly withdraw affectively and/or cognitively from our patients. In so doing, we violate implicit professional norms but keep that violation to ourselves.

Here are some anecdotal examples of minor and more serious delinquencies. All are undisguised and reported with permission. Some were described by patients; others by analysts about themselves. They include: Making a note to oneself about a forgotten task; adding to a grocery list; planning an event; filing or painting nails; combing hair; putting on makeup; surfing the web; eating a snack; skimming magazines or journals; checking email; buying airline tickets online; reading correspondence; pumping breast milk; watching a sports scoreboard online; writing patients' bills; deliberately cutting a session short by a minute or two; charging for a missed session during the analyst's own vacation of which the patient was unaware; and quietly going to the bathroom during a telephone session while muting the phone.

Additional delinquencies became common during Covid. Most involve multitasking while on screen—e.g., checking email, reading and replying to texts, surfing the web, or secretly doing something out of the camera's scope (putting on hand cream, removing one's shoes, eating). All the therapists I spoke to were certain that their patients were entirely oblivious. True? Denial? I'm not sure, but it's rare for patients to address the breach with the analyst.

Another group of misdemeanors are engaged in openly during face-to-face sessions. These include taking long phone calls, using a treatment hour to satisfy personal needs (e.g., talking at length to a patient about a matter of personal concern or asking a patient to recommend physicians, stocks, discount clothing stores, restaurants, etc.). One colleague reported that a patient's previous analyst regularly ate dinner during their sessions until the patient exploded with the comment, "What is this, a fucking picnic?"

In contrast to hidden misdemeanors, open breaches are more clearly located within the relational domain. Emerging out of implicit aspects of the treatment relationship, they may represent a form of unconscious communication with the patient. When the analyst acts openly, it ought to be easier for the patient to respond directly to a breach. Yet this happens relatively rarely, perhaps because there's a silent pressure on the patient *not* to notice, or anyway address, what the analyst is doing. Excluded from therapeutic discourse, open breaches may, in fact, function like secret ones.

Describing his previous treatment, Samuel mentioned that his analyst frequently ate a sandwich as they talked. Samuel hadn't been consciously bothered by this and, probably in response to my surprised expression, added that his analyst had asked if he minded, and he had said no. Consciously, Samuel enjoyed these dinner sessions because he was left with the feeling that things were "comfy" between them. Samuel not only didn't object to his therapist's dinner hour, he enjoyed his "special place" symbolically embodied in these dinner sessions.

But there was more to it than met the eye. Despite his apparent consent to this breach of etiquette, Samuel was, in fact, quite *unfree* in that interaction. Samuel felt compelled to comply with, and not react negatively to, his analyst's desire to eat. In going along with his therapist's request, Samuel placed himself (and was placed) in a compliant position, a pattern of relatedness reminiscent of Samuel's relationship with both parents, an experience that had left Samuel with a major difficulty with self-assertion. His analyst's apparent obliviousness to all this reinforced Samuel's chronic sense that his needs were less important than those of the other. Despite considerable work around issues of self-effacement, the dyad excluded this theme as it played out between them; they established a context of apparent ease that was contingent on Samuel's participation as a compliant partner. This complicity left Samuel silenced and passive once again.

It's difficult to ascertain the relative weight of the analyst's conscious self-interest and his unconscious participation in this reenactment. But given that the analyst focused on Samuel's needs at other times, I suspect that a key motivational factor involved personal need—in this case, hunger—leading the analyst to override what he knew about Samuel and recreate an exploitative interaction.

On another level, Samuel may have assimilated a different but equally troublesome message; perhaps his analyst had difficulty meeting his own needs—after all, he regularly deprived himself of a dinner break. Did Samuel identify with his analyst's implicit self-deprivation, reinforcing Samuel's relational pattern? Alternatively, did Samuel's analyst unconsciously identify with *Samuel's* difficulty taking for himself, enacting and reversing that difficulty by simultaneously eating and working?

## Enactments, crimes, and object relatedness

It's not easy to delineate the boundary between enactments, delinquencies, and serious analytic breaches. These categories are more overlapping than distinct; what constitutes a misdemeanor to us may feel like a crime to our patient or colleague, or vice versa. Further, such distinctions can be self-serving; by attributing our actions to relational dynamics and reenactments, we avoid confronting unpleasant realities that collide with our self-image as caring and committed analysts. But when we label an action a crime, we defensively embrace a rigid, moralistic position that can foreclose, rather than open, the process.

Enactments that emerge in the emotional or erotic heat of an analytic encounter are ubiquitous. These breaches are usually briefly, rather than permanently, destabilizing. By addressing previously dissociated relational dynamics, the work deepens. But major boundary violations involve very different issues. When analysts violate basic professional norms by, for example, sleeping with patients, stealing from them, or otherwise exploiting them for personal gain, the treatment relationship will likely be permanently destroyed. Major boundary violations negate or deliberately exploit the patient's subjectivity and vulnerability. The analyst may be confronted with legal suit, ethical censure, or both.

Gabbard and Lester (1995), detailing the early history of boundary violations beginning with Freud, describe both sexual and nonsexual transgressions. They note that boundary violations typically reflect a slide down a slippery slope wherein the analyst's emotional involvement gradually erodes awareness of the patient's vulnerability and needs.

## Delinquencies: The analyst as a subject

I locate delinquencies along a continuum marked by major boundary violations at one pole and enactments on the other. In contrast to the spontaneous affective eruption that typically characterizes enactments, most misdemeanors are deliberately committed and contain less affective charge; the analyst isn't engaged in reverie (Ogden, 1994, 1997) but in purposeful inattention. In this sense, delinquencies aren't unlike more serious boundary violations. However, where major boundary violations involve explicit exploitation of the patient, misdemeanors usually reflect the analyst's attentional and affective *withdrawal* from the arena of patient need into a state of solipsistic subjecthood so that the analyst becomes the single subject in the room.

Analysts are especially vulnerable to committing infractions in treatments characterized by ongoing chronic boredom or emotional disengagement. By momentarily removing herself from the treatment experience, the analyst does something for herself, perhaps in an unconscious attempt at self-restoration.

Self-involved patients tend to be unaware of the analyst's removal *and* of their own impact (Bach, 1985). Whether through selective inattention (Sullivan, 1954) or by leaving such experiences unformulated (D. B. Stern, 1997), the patient ignores/brackets whatever might disrupt the experience of attunement (Jacobs, 1991; Slochower, 1996c, 2014d).

I wonder if it's precisely the *absence* of intense emotional demands on the patient's part that creates room for the analyst to move this way. This retreat from the relational field is, surely, an abandonment of the patient and the analytic task. Still, misdemeanors are less abusive than analytic crimes (or delinquencies committed in face-to-face sessions) because the latter transform the patient from subject to object in an explicitly exploitative way[1].

## Our misbehavior and our professional self-image

The analytic community shares a consensual vision of the treatment frame that certainly doesn't include analytic misdemeanors. Yet, while the types of breaches and the frequency with which they're committed are highly variable, it's my sense that only the unusual or perhaps very young analyst is completely innocent in this regard. The bulk of ethical lapses aren't committed by psychopathic practitioners (Celenza & Gabbard, 2003). More typically, misdemeanors represent circumscribed moments within a given treatment that stand in stark contrast to an analyst's ordinarily high level of responsible engagement and solid analytic work.

---

1  Sue Grand (2000) illustrates this in her discussion of human malevolence.

Because most analysts are enormously invested in their self-image as caring and committed professionals, even small professional breaches pose a threat to self-esteem. When therapists sneakily transgress their own professional standards, colleagues and supervisors can seem like the moral police whose judgment must be sidestepped. So it's hardly surprising that misdemeanors are seldom talked about, let alone brought into supervision; indeed, even minor professional breaches tend to be sequestered both from self-examination and analytic discourse and result in a quasi-conscious disavowal on analyst's *and* patient's part. On those occasions when a delinquency is detected, analysts may commit a second breach by rationalizing (or lying) to cover up their action. Ultimately, such disavowal invites more egregious misdemeanors that traverse the permeable boundary between delinquencies and serious analytic crimes.

Analysts aren't alone in their resistance to examining these moments of professional failure; most patients find it extremely difficult to address them directly, perhaps because doing so exposes both members of the dyad to the reality of the lapse. Hidden misdemeanors appear to shield the patient from the analyst's actions; most of the analysts with whom I spoke felt certain their patients were unaware of their inattention. In those few cases where the analyst's infraction was exposed, patients expressed surprisingly little distress. It's impossible, of course, to know whether these muted responses reflected disavowal, an attempt to relieve the analyst's guilt, anxiety about expressing anger, or other dynamics.

Let's return to Dr. M. With both embarrassment and worry about my censorious reaction but with strikingly little curiosity about her behavior, she described her magazine sneaking. I agreed that magazines shouldn't be read during telephone sessions but I asked whether we could look at her action with curiosity rather than censure. Her patient, Mr. J, was an earnest young man who had difficulty accessing his emotional life. Mr. J's intellectualized style led him to drone a bit, and Dr. M sometimes struggled against boredom during their sessions; this was especially true during telephone contacts. They had agreed to use the phone to maintain continuity during his extended business trips and, consciously at least, Dr. M felt comfortable with this arrangement[2].

---

2  It's interesting to consider whether the use of the telephone and Zoom increases the risk of enacting delinquencies. When we use the telephone or computer, do we unconsciously feel less like an analyst, freed from professional constrictions and obligations?

I wondered aloud if Dr. M read magazines to cope with Mr. J's emotional withdrawal out of an unconscious sense of hopelessness about contacting him. Was she expressing disowned resentment toward Mr. J for his frequent absences by removing herself emotionally? Dr. M felt especially deprived of contact in the absence of the visual stimulation of the in-person session; perhaps she had responded to this deprivation by turning to magazines to fill in the missing visual element.

Feeling we had done a good piece of supervisory work I was surprised to hear Dr. M say with much embarrassment that she doubted that her action could be explained in this way because she *regularly* looked through magazines during phone sessions with many patients. She looked forward to phone sessions because they gave her a chance to relax a bit. Dr. M was peripherally aware she was doing something wrong but had avoided thinking about her actions.

Thus, despite the unique aspects of Dr. M's response to Mr. J, her misdemeanors also involved chronic expressions of opportunism. Dr. M regularly took advantage of telephone sessions or patients' use of the couch to look through magazines and, in other small ways, satisfy herself while still playing the role of good analyst. When a therapeutic hour left her feeling bored, deprived, or otherwise disengaged, Dr. M made use of her hidden position to "steal" something for herself. It's noteworthy that Dr. M didn't commit these breaches on the phone with more difficult or distressed patients who "demanded" her attention. Here, her ordinary good-analyst self took over; sustained by the affective contact and intellectual stimulation of the work, she felt no wish to retreat[3].

Acknowledging this for the first time, Dr. M expressed intense guilt, shame, and anxiety about what she identified as a failure of professionalism and an abandonment of her patients. Trying to help her leave judgment aside, I focused on a heretofore disavowed sense of depletion and strain that pervaded Dr. M's working life. Financial stress had led her to take on a maximum number of patient hours. Dr. M wondered whether her "easier" patients recognized how much difficulty she had had openly taking what she needed and "allowed" her these periods of emotional respite. Dr. M was

---

3  A colleague commented that Dr. M's willingness to reveal herself within the supervisory context was unusual. I agree. This supervisory relationship, *outside* the institute training framework, probably played a role in "permitting" her to take this chance.

also aware there wasn't much she could do about the ongoing strain in her life. Ultimately, she decided to stop doing telephone sessions except in real emergencies. Now conscious of her tendency to withdraw from Mr. J, Dr. M gradually intensified her emotional involvement with him and addressed the subtle enactment that had been taking place[4].

Dr. M's misdemeanors reflected the press of her own unmet needs and seemed to coalesce largely outside the relational arena. Not infrequently, however, delinquencies emerge out of relational dynamics. After hearing me give a talk on this subject, Dr. O confessed that he regularly ended sessions with his most "impossible" patient a few minutes early because "I can't wait for the session to be over." Interestingly, Dr. O's patient didn't seem to notice these early endings (or perhaps was equally eager to be rid of his analyst).

Dr. O knew he was cheating his patient out of his full time but wasn't aware of its underlying dynamics. Dr. O deeply doubted his therapeutic capacity and tended to rely on reassurance from his patients. This very difficult patient failed to provide needed reassurance; by ending their hours early, Dr. O's disavowed self-doubt found expression. What first appeared to be a rather high-handed disregard for his patient's right to a full treatment hour turned out to be driven by far more complex dynamics.

To some extent, misdemeanors are personally and relationally defined; each analytic relationship shapes the treatment boundaries and rules of engagement a bit differently. Yet despite these subjective and contextual factors, there's an overarching ethical standard—an analytic ideal—to which we aspire.

Some types of analytic behavior that we now regard with disapproval were viewed as unremarkable during earlier periods in the history of psychoanalysis. Analysts knitted, crocheted, allowed dogs and cats in the consulting room, supervised, socialized with patients, and so on. Today, we mostly don't. But in most other respects, the psychoanalytic ideal has loosened with time. Even pre-Covid, some of us conducted telephone or FaceTime/Zoom sessions when patients were traveling. Today, nearly all

---

4 Dr. M decided not to confess her misdemeanor to Mr. J. Although her guilty feelings would have been alleviated, Dr. M worried that her patient would feel betrayed and attack himself for his failure to keep her attention. In subsequent months, Dr. M listened for evidence that Mr. J had subliminally been aware of this period of inattention. She found none.

of us have incorporated technology into therapeutic process; it's been our only alternative.

Our emphasis on the *analyst as a person* has further shifted our view of the treatment relationship in a less formalized direction. We understand professional breaches through the lens of relational dynamics; we study what's being replayed rather than merely condemning the analyst for her misbehavior.

## Acting out, corruption, or burnout?

Analytic delinquencies often reflect burnout, overwork, or intensified personal strain. When we're driven by professional interest, need, or greed to see more patients and work longer days, a sense of inner pressure is nearly inevitable. And when we don't allow ourselves, or are unable, to create other venues for personal restoration, emotional or physical depletion can become chronic. By committing a misdemeanor, the analyst attempts to secretly take something for herself, something she hasn't allowed herself to take openly—for example, time, or social contact.

The asymmetrical nature of the analytic relationship (Aron, 1996) heightens the impact of these delinquencies; in committing delinquencies, we exploit our power and expose the malignant underbelly to the analytic position Hoffman (1998) describes. Usually, that dynamic remains unconscious, but occasionally, it's deliberate.

Rationalizing that "all analysts misbehave," Dr. F seemed not to experience guilt when he ignored basic therapeutic rules. Consciously rejecting his professional ideal, Dr. F's actions became increasingly psychopathic and rationalized. When he found himself threatened with a lawsuit by a patient (he had asked the patient to invest money for him), he gave up his license rather than face the prospect of a legal battle. Only then did he confront his abandonment of professional ethics.

More often, delinquencies represent a response to disavowed needs. Dr. V chronically ignored his own depleted emotional state while complaining that his patients "sucked him dry." Dr. V hated those patients who remained in need when he felt he had little left to give; he couldn't make peace with the discrepancy between his own emotionally compromised position and his patients' more comfortable circumstances. That hatred found expression in symbolic acts of theft—of time and attention—from them. Bitter and deprived, Dr. V rationalized his actions as a legitimate response to the difficult straits he was in. His personal difficulties resulted in a disidentification with—and corruption of—his analytic ideal. Cynically dismissing his professional commitment and the value of psychoanalysis itself, Dr. V's capacity to sustain a professional stance dissolved until his behavior actually became corrupt (Chessick, 1994).

Most analysts never flagrantly violate their professional role in these ways. But we also don't acknowledge the ubiquity of small professional breaches. Indeed, my younger colleagues uniformly responded with outrage and shock to the idea that analysts commit these acts. They ascribed misdemeanors to burnout and a loss of ethical standards; several declared that they would terminate their analysis were their analysts ever to commit even the smallest breach. Yet most of the older analysts I spoke with responded with recognition and sometimes amusement to this material and spontaneously added other examples of professional misdemeanors to my list[5]. Some seemed to view their misbehavior as a rebellion, more or less conscious, against their own theoretical model, while others saw their actions as selfishly motivated. Although I surmise that shame and guilt lay beneath their amusement, I also heard a tendency to rationalize. Had a layer of cynicism infiltrated their professionalism in a way that hadn't yet compromised the idealism of younger therapists?

## The analyst's countertransference and the analyst's compromise

Some delinquencies are driven by factors unique to particular treatment configurations. The analyst reacts to ongoing relational dynamics with an intensified sense of need and disregards or negates her commitment to the analytic ideal.

This isn't altogether surprising; although most of us derive considerable gratification from our therapeutic role, it's equally true that we sometimes feel quite deprived—concretely or symbolically—as we attempt to remain present, to set aside our personal agenda, preoccupations, and emotional states for multiple analytic hours across the day. The struggle to "be there" for every patient inevitably collides with our needs. Small delinquencies may be motivated by an unconscious effort to balance these two desires—

---

5 This "dark side" of the analytic frame may be expressed, for example, in a potentially exploitative request to publish material about a particular patient.

a rather unsatisfactory compromise between the wish to be a good analyst and the desire to satisfy personal needs. I suspect that most misdemeanors contain this element of inner negotiation on the analyst's part (S. A. Pizer, 1998). The attempt to balance or regulate conflicting needs is both camou-flaged *and* embodied in acts of delinquency.

Some years ago, while working on this essay, I caught myself com-mitting a momentary lapse that illustrates one of these moments of inner negotiation. I suspect that many, perhaps most, of these negotiations go unnoticed; I suspect that this breach would have remained so were I not writing about misdemeanors.

Over the weekend, I had found an old photo of my now grown-up daughter, about 10 at the time. The picture showed her smiling hugely and looking utterly adorable, and I slipped it into a pile on my desk, planning to put it into an album later. During a session with a quiet, hard working analytic patient who's engaged with me in a low-key way, I impulsively picked up the photo and smiled at my daughter's aliveness and youthful beauty. For perhaps 10 seconds I was suffused with a sense of warmth and personal pleasure as I returned to an earlier time and imagined cud-dling her and sharing her joy. This was stolen pleasure. I briefly but quasi-deliberately removed myself from my patient, although I didn't lose track of his process.

Had I unconsciously used this moment of contact with my intensely alive daughter to counterbalance the very quiet, sad, and on some level, less gratifying emotionality between my patient and me? But this explanation implies that my action emerged purely out of my own need state; it ignores the element of reenactment that likely was embedded within it. Like my patient's parents, I became momentarily preoccupied; he didn't hold my attention as he had not held theirs.

On one level, my withdrawal might represent a form of reverie (Ogden, 1994) from which I emerged with a renewed awareness of the treatment dynamics and an intensified engagement with my patient. I want to empha-size, though, the *deliberateness* with which I turned to that photo in contrast to the more unconscious flavor of enactments or the peripheral cognitive and emotional phenomena Ogden describes, wherein we *find* our attention wandering elsewhere. In this instance, I briefly withdrew from a difficult emotional engagement and sought a simpler and more joyous moment with my daughter.

Brief lapses such as these are probably ubiquitous. It's when those efforts fail in more major ways that we're vulnerable to committing major breaches of the analytic contract.

## Misdemeanors as rebellion

Frankel (2003) proposed that a subversive element may be embedded in misdemeanors. By refusing to comply with a rigidly held ideal, we preserve our right to make our own judgments; we choose which rules of practice we follow and those we reject.

Subversion is a tricky concept; it implies rebellion *against* authority. When we attempt to undercut authority, we don't so much step out of the power dynamic as reverse it; the controlled becomes the controller. The alternative to submission isn't necessarily opposition; the latter may side-step a genuine search for self-definition, for a position that's our own, integrated, not simply a reaction *against* the ideal.

Bernstein (2003) suggests that some analytic theories heighten our vulnerability to committing misdemeanors more than others. She highlights the pressure that Winnicottian models place on analysts. An idealization of the maternal (analytic) position might lead us to commit delinquencies that express those aspects of our self-interest incompatible with a maternal role.

But this doesn't mean that if we allow ourselves to be less maternal we wouldn't commit misdemeanors. Because there's an obverse problem. Kleinian or Lacanian analysts (or, for that matter, interpersonal or relational analysts) might feel required to *resist* gratifying their patients' apparent need for a maternal response. Might they not find themselves in a different, yet ultimately similar, kind of conundrum? Couldn't the struggle to set aside a *wish* to express maternal feelings provoke its own delinquency? Might our breach be a response to emotional deprivation or the desire for more affect or warmth than the prescribed role permits?

It's probably impossible to resolve the tension between the analytic ideal and our self-interest by subscribing to a specific theoretical model. Inherent in every theory are rules we may find difficult to follow. Different theories minimize and maximize our opportunity to express aspects of our personhood within the work; they tilt us toward some misdemeanors and away from others. But no theory provides us with a solution to the collision of self-interest and our professional ideal.

## The moral imperative and the moralizing analyst

Activities like magazine reading, which shift our cognitive focus, limit our capacity to be emotionally present; rationalizing the lapse sets us on a course that may lead to disaster. After all, we're paid to pay attention. Yes, we're vulnerable to reverie and other kinds of unconscious moments of inattention, but we're really not supposed to deliberately use our patients' time to meet our own needs.

And here's my conundrum: By naming our delinquencies, I'm likely to arouse a guilty reaction in the reader. Not a great result. Guilt provokes avoidance, denial, sometimes intense self-reproach. None is likely to open reflective space. *Is* it possible to explore the dynamics of our delinquencies without intensifying a censorious superego voice that sternly reminds us to behave? Or will this superego element lead us to externalize, minimize, or disavow our misbehavior? Will you read this chapter as moralizing despite my attempt to engage curiosity rather than self-reproach?

I'm advocating a posture of self-reflection but *not* of self-judgment. We *need* ideals; they derive from an underlying moral theory that proscribes certain kinds of behavior. Implicit is a "common ethical ground" (Wallerstein, 1990) that we share. Professional ethics largely transcend the particulars of different psychoanalytic theories; they emphasize patients' vulnerability and our obligation to meet their needs within the codes of other health professionals (e.g., the Hippocratic oath).

I use the words misdemeanors and delinquencies, then, *not* in a legalistic sense but because they characterize analytic *self-experience*. We embrace an ethical code of conduct and are uncomfortably aware of times that we've reversed that basic commitment. We confront our *own* censorious voices when we break the rules and hide bits of what we do from ourselves, our patients, or our colleagues.

There's a basic therapeutic position that cuts across theoretical divides. It reflects our commitment, within the treatment hour, to putting our patients' needs first and addressing whatever resistances interfere with our doing so. Even if self-regulatory in intent, some of the misdemeanors we commit go way beyond this aim and take us *away* from our patients. If we focus solely on how those actions humanize us, embed an enactment, or protect the treatment, don't we run the risk of sidestepping their troublesome, even destructive, impact?

## The analyst's idealized responsiveness

There's something ironic about the notion that to do good analytic work we must be present as full and feeling persons while consistently using our humanity in the service of our patients' needs. And while the past decade has both humanized and softened our professional ideal, it's inevitable that the press of our own needs will be insufficiently met when we're working. While individual analysts respond to different dimensions of the analytic ideal with a feeling of increased strain, we all contend with that pressure during periods of personal life stress, illness, or other crises.

Winnicott (1947) suggested that the analyst expresses her selfishness or hatred of the patient in symbolic ways, for example, in the strict ending of the hour. He believed that this expression supported the treatment and the analyst and allowed her to work more effectively.

But what if these symbolic expressions of personal need aren't enough? *Are* we capable of remaining focused on our patient for much of the working day in a manner more complete than is required, perhaps, in any other profession? Unless we own and consciously struggle with our greed, sense of deprivation, or selfishness (Kraemer, 1996; Slavin & Kriegman, 1998), it's nearly inevitable that those feelings will be expressed illicitly.

Delinquencies disrupt the treatment contract and represent a real failure of the analytic function. Yet they also reflect our abiding and immutable humanity, the limits of our ability to fully suspend personal needs in the context of a requirement that we do so.

The analytic ideal contains a disregard for those dimensions of our humanness that are *not* integral to the treatment relationship. Misdemeanors are ubiquitous precisely because we find it so difficult to acknowledge and work with the clash between our very human selfishness and the still excessive demands of this "impossible profession."

We need to contend with this paradox. To simultaneously embrace the analytic ideal, its collision with our own very real and limiting humanity, and our commitment to sustaining an ongoing struggle against the abandonment of that ideal.

# Chapter 7

# Ghosts that haunt

Isn't it odd. Psychoanalytic theories have their origins in ideas about sexuality's psychic elements; we write prodigiously about erotics in the transference and countertransference. We speak about the reality of erotics in the consulting room; about the actuality of sexual boundary violations (relatively rarely). Yet it's fact, not rumor, that there are virtually no psychoanalytic communities in which sexual boundary violations between analyst and patient didn't—and don't—occur.

The shadow of sexual boundary violations has followed us across generations; victims become perpetrators who reverse and reenact the trauma they experienced. The rest of us are witnesses, albeit indirect ones. Unsurprisingly, most of us remain publicly silent, though often privately distressed about what we either know or have heard. It's time we talked.

There's a huge literature on the dynamics of the boundary violator and the victim (e.g., Celenza, 2007, 2017, 2021; Celenza & Gabbard, 2003; Dimen, 2011; Gabbard, 1995a, 1995b, 2014, 2017; Gabbard & Lester, 1995; Gabbard, Peltz, & the COPE Study Group, 2001; Grand, 2010, 2017b; Margolis, 1997; Pepper, 2014; B. Pizer, 2000; Sandler & Godley, 2004). Here, though, I focus on a shadow phenomenon, on what happens—psychologically speaking—to those of us who are *not* directly involved.

## What do we do with—and about—what we know?

Our field has been plagued by sexual boundary violations since its beginnings. Loewald (1960), borrowing the term "ghosts" from Freud (1953) (and indirectly from Homer), noted that violations have an impact that's at once insidious, unnameable, and profound (Honig & Barron, 2013). These ghosts hover at the edge of our psychoanalytic institutes, coloring—indeed tainting—our feelings about the profession, institute, and sometimes our

DOI: 10.4324/9781032691534-11

colleagues. Popping into the clinical encounter, awareness of the violator becomes a "not me" element that disturbs, disrupts, and occasionally derails us. I think this is true both for those who have personal relationships with the victim or perpetrator *and* for those who don't (Slochower, 2017b, 2017c).

We psychoanalysts may represent a clinical/theoretical Tower of Babel in many respects, but one thing binds us together: Despite our commitment to protecting our patients, analysts and therapists have been engaging in sexual boundary violations since this field began. While we're enormously disturbed by this, we've done little to address it; in fact, we've mostly colluded to keep it out of sight, if not out of mind. While we don't quite fall prey to the kind of malignant dissociative contagion Grand (2000) speaks about, we tend to deal with what cannot be encompassed by retreating from it.

What's more disturbing than learning that a colleague is having sex with a patient? Not only is our trust in the violator threatened, but the field's integrity also is called into question. Our need to protect ourselves, our institute, and the larger psychoanalytic community pulls us to foreclose what we suspect and how we feel about it. Overriding a sense of moral outrage, we deny, even dissociate what we know.

It's not surprising that sexual boundary violations recur across generations; their victims—like victims of other trauma—are especially vulnerable to reenacting, in reverse, the assault they experienced. Too often, the victim is left feeling abandoned, shamed, or blamed. Left alone to metabolize the experience, she rarely has access to a recognizing group that can act as witness on her behalf and/or against the perpetrator.

## Personal encounters

I was a young candidate in the early 1980s when I had my first indirect encounter with sexual boundary violations. A good friend, in analysis with a respected male analyst 20 years her senior, confided that he had been making explicit sexual advances toward her. She shut them down but continued the treatment, remaining silent both with him and about him.

If she had been traumatized by this experience, she kept it to herself. Her matter-of-fact silence confused me; I couldn't assimilate, much less articulate, how I felt about all this. Instead, I filed away what I knew and held it in a space apart. This was, I thought, most likely a single incident in the career of a widely esteemed analyst. What would be gained by creating trouble for someone to whom so many were devoted? There seemed to be no way to hold his talent in tension with his transgressions and I sidelined the latter.

It turned out that my friend had been far from alone in her experience. Rumors—some vague, others specific—began to surface, communicated in whispers intermingled with both horror and prurient pleasure. My friend's analyst and another well-known senior person had breached sexual boundaries with both supervisees and patients. Decades later, we know that these were neither rumors nor isolated occurrences.

But things stopped there. The perpetrators were never publicly named, and no actions were taken. The wider community was left disturbed and mystified.

### Should we tell?

Perhaps. But we usually don't.

What informs the decision to report or not report a sexual boundary violation? Do we feel complicit, guilty both about our silence *and* about our wish to tell? Are we only a few steps away from the brink ourselves? To name a transgressor may stimulate our own bad-analyst feeling (Epstein, 1999), anxiety, and guilt about our misbehavior or wish to misbehave. Does whistleblowing feel like an act of aggression or duplicity rather than something done on behalf of the victim and larger community?

Our need to remain silent often goes beyond an allegiance to the violator: We have an investment in protecting our community and in affirming our professional ideal, an ideal that collides with the reality of having sex with a patient. To make matters worse, reporting a suspected or known boundary violation may damage our community's place in the wider professional world. Will we disrupt, even dismantle, the experience of those analysands, supervisees, and students who were, in fact, helped by the violator analyst? Will we provoke public skepticism about psychoanalysis as a profession and contribute to its demise?

What if naming names triggers excessive punitiveness on the part of administrators and the larger community? What if we're responsible for destroying someone's career? And then there's our own vulnerability: Will we become the object of retaliation, if not by the perpetrator then by those who surround and want to protect him? There are so many good reasons not to act.

For some, sociopolitical factors are embedded in our silence. Those who came of age in political times and places demanding compliance and prohibiting dissent may remain especially reluctant to become "tat-tletales." We identify with the underdog; we refuse to become inform-ants. Indeed, many of us are identified with the ethical autonomy inherent in that avoidance. It's not an autonomy that easily moves us to whistleblowing.

In the United States, our reluctance may reflect the traumatic shadow of the McCarthy era, a period when resistance to authority carried considerable risk. When informants accused my father of being a com-munist during the McCarthy era, he pleaded the Fifth Amendment (the American Constitutional right to avoid self-incrimination) because he didn't want to be forced to name his communist colleagues. He was nevertheless fired from his academic position at Brooklyn College. The case eventually ended up in the Supreme Court, where he won and was reinstated, many years after the fact. Unsurprisingly, I grew up acutely aware of the dangers of tattling. And my experience is far from unique (see Lyons, 2014).

## Whose erotic fantasy is it anyway?

There's another dynamic layer that may inform our silence—it's the need to sidestep our excited response to a colleague's sexual breach. The erotic horror (Kumin, 1985–1986) we experience may embody our own vulner-ability to sexual feelings in the countertransference. After all, who among us has never committed a small boundary violation or permitted them-selves a sexual fantasy about a patient? Who has never harbored hostile fantasies about a colleague? And while most of us have never engaged in sexual boundary crossings, I bet nearly all of us have had moments when we wished we could.

Reporting a boundary violation allows us to symbolically locate "bad-ness" out there where it doesn't threaten our own good-analyst feeling. We get the charge of an erotically colored shocking story while remaining above the fray. But this element of titillation isn't uncomplicated. Gossiping about a colleague's sexual acting out likely evokes both shame and pleasure in us—responses to trauma that meld with a more ordinary erotic excitement and leave us feeling at once ashamed and affectively elevated. Lurking beneath may be grief, identification with the victim, anger, and a sense of powerlessness. No wonder we remain silent.

When sexual boundary violations come to light, public discussions occur infrequently; rarer still is there a vehicle for exploration or reconciliation at the individual or group level. Whispered gossip has so often been our only relief/release. Is our gossip a kind of emotional masturbation—stimulating but lacking a climax or finality that would contain and settle things?

## The traumatic element

If we ourselves were/are victims of betrayal—sexual or not; early or recent—our response to a current sexual boundary violation will likely be vastly intensified. Assimilating it procedurally rather than consciously, we remain frozen and mute, unable to articulate our anxiety, outrage, or identificatory sense of trauma. Our silence doesn't reflect indifference, however. It's a PTSD response to the nearly unthinkable, combined with a profound sense of helplessness. We don't know what to say, whom to tell, or what to do. Deeply disturbed, we become immobilized.

The fact that sexual breaches are frequently committed by those with professional power only intensifies the traumatic element. Often, the violator has gravitas: He[1] may even have been a psychoanalytic "great," someone we idealized. Like the father in the 1950s American TV serial *Father Knows Best*, we want to believe he *does* know best. How could he have ignored, indeed flaunted, our code of professional ethics, acted as if the rules didn't apply to him? His behavior shakes up, even dismantles, our professional ideal and we become both distressed and disillusioned.

## Dismantled idealizations

Most of us want—and need—to believe in the field's (and our own) curative potential, in our capacity to set aside the excesses of personal need in the best interest of our patient. The perpetrator may be a revered mentor, writer, former (or present) supervisor, teacher, or analyst and our idealization of

---

1 I refer to the violator as "he" in this chapter. While sexual boundary violations occur between female analyst–male patient pairs and between gay analytic couples of both genders, most transgressions are committed in male analyst–female patient constellations, and it's here that I focus.

him leads us to half rationalize. Perhaps his therapeutic brilliance allowed him to ignore boundaries without compromising his healing capacity. Perhaps he really *was* acting in the best interest of the patient, at least most of the time. Were we to assimilate the reality of what actually happened, it would shatter that idealization (Slochower, 2011b, 2014a, 2014c, 2015b, 2018a).

If our idealization enables the violator, it comes at a high personal price: Abandoning our own sense of ethical agency—a sensibility with both personal and professional derivations—we fail to name what we know. We become collaborators—passive participants in something we abhor. An exaggerated asymmetry effectively ties our own hands and renders us smaller, less wise, less aware than we are, while elevating the stature of the idealized other. Certainly, the actual violator bears primary ethical responsibility for what he does, but we enable him by virtue of our silence. Our idealization thus has a malignant underbelly: It obfuscates what we need not to see and not to know. It invites our passive participation in the sexual breach and in this sense, it renders us complicit.

Yet our idealizations aren't something we can do without. We need to believe in our mentors and in the field of psychoanalysis. Our ideals remind us of the importance of professional ethics and integrity, self-reflectivity, the honesty of the field (Ackerman, 2020). In some respects, ideals represent a wedge against delinquencies, against what Hirsch (2008) called "coasting in the countertransference." Steadying us in the face of clinical uncertainty, our ideals inspire and sustain us; they give us something against which to evaluate ourselves. And they ought to serve as a barrier to both sexual and nonsexual boundary violations.

But they usually don't. If anything, our ideals have made it nearly impossible for us to face either their excesses or their vulnerability to collapse. Too often, the space between our ideals and actuality silences us; it invites compartmentalization, denial, even disavowal. I quote: "It's not possible that he had sex with the patient, it's a nasty rumor perpetrated by those who envy him"; "She wasn't a patient; she was just a supervisee"; "It was a single incident, not such a big deal." At other times, we find more complex—but equally troublesome—ways of rationalizing what happened: "Sometimes people really fall in love. The patient is his age and they're both in the field; they made a mature, conscious decision to move the relationship into a different arena." Or even, shocking in its cynicism/naïveté, "Come on. It's not as if he raped her."

When evidence of harm makes rationalization impossible—for example, when the analyst is decades older than the patient or when the patient falls apart or presses charges—we may move disavowal in a different direction. We maintain our idealization by blaming—really pathologizing—the victim and simultaneously emphasizing the analyst's innocence and benign intentions: "The patient is borderline, unbelievably seductive. I bet she hallucinated half of it, turned his kindly touch into a sexual moment"; "He thought he was helping her, and she seduced him into playing out her abuse history. He's naïve but really, he's a good guy. And she's extraordinarily self-destructive."

Despite the denial embedded in these idealizations (and an implicit denigration of the patient), there's often a bit of truth. Patient victims frequently bring their own abuse history into the treatment relationship; those dynamics contribute to its sexual denouement and make it easier for us to blame her. Adding to our confusion is the fact that violators are rarely guilty of cold, calculated abuse. Most are probably not psychopaths, and most aren't entirely defined by their actions; they may be brilliant writers or may do sensitive, skilled therapeutic work with other patients.

Analysts—themselves vulnerable to fantasy—sometimes lose track of their own need or wish for intimacy, rescue, or idealized love. Sexual violations are typically the endpoint of a slow slide down a slippery slope with a particular patient—not with all patients. Should we utterly blacken the name and destroy the reputation of someone who also resides outside the realm of analytic failure?

The desire to protect the violator's stature reverberates at a more abstract level because the wish to preserve our professional ideal collides with the need to call a spade a spade. What if "telling" damages our community's place in the wider professional world? What if we disrupt, even dismantle, the experience of those analysands, supervisees, and students who were, in fact, helped by the analyst? In declaring that the emperor has no clothes, will we take down our kingdom?

To further complicate things, whistleblowing is its own wild card. What if naming names triggers excessive punitiveness on the part of ethics committees and the larger community (Celenza, 2007)? What if we do more harm than good? Will we be punished for telling, if not by the perpetrator then by those who surround and want to protect him? To make matters worse, often (though not always) the violator is someone with professional power; we fear his (and his supporters') capacity to retaliate.

We're silent because we're scared. Our anxiety may even make us doubt what we know.

All kinds of legal constraints coalesce with these personal anxieties and shut us down. In the United States, state law defines whether anyone other than the victim patient can report a sexual violation; in many states, those who "know" via hearsay or even direct communications cannot initiate action; only the victim can file a complaint. Furthermore, both the whistleblower and the institute itself are vulnerable to libel suits when names are named; those in positions of administrative power are silenced by their own legal counsel. Too frequently, our hands are tied; there's nothing concrete we can do with what we know or suspect. Scared, fearful of making trouble, feeling impotent, we become doubtful. *Are* we sure? After all, we weren't there. What if we're wrong? Helpless, frustrated, we sideline what we know.

When reality becomes undeniable and we're confronted with what we cannot exclude, our idealization shatters, replaced by bitter disillusionment. "He's a sleazeball." "He's losing it." "He thinks with his dick." We effectively excommunicate the analyst, eject him from our psychic and literal midst. In part we do this because the analyst's behavior has, in fact, been reprehensible and deserving of ostracism. But I think another dynamic is often at work here: As we denigrate the analyst, we simultaneously find a way to protect our idealization by relocating it elsewhere: "He's not a real analyst"; "He's no hero of mine; Dr. X, on the other hand, would never behave this way. It's he I emulate."

## Our theory and our boundaries

Those who commit major boundary violations often justify their actions by invoking a clinical theory that apparently rationalizes their rejection of the ordinary analytic frame. The patient's vulnerability and need, sexual or emotional inhibition, require it.

The breach often begins when the analyst responds to the patient's trauma history and the intensity of baby needs with a sense that extraordinary measures are required. Rescue fantasies merge with underlying grandiosity and disavowed rage, precipitating a gradual slippage toward sexual transgression, a slippage apparently supported by the analyst's theory of clinical action (Gabbard, personal communication, 2017).

At times, the analyst uses his theory to justify a boundary breach. Here's an example: A young woman's Freudian analyst regularly masturbated her to orgasm in the name of activating her "dead libido." His theoretical investment in the power of drives was used perversely as a rationalization for sexual acting out. This analyst's grandiosity, supported by his stature in the community, protected him from scrutiny, let alone censure. Another patient, in therapy with an interpersonal analyst, told me that the therapist frequently took her to lunch, after which he kissed and fondled her. The therapist seemed to believe that free social/sexual interaction would help his shy and self-deprecating patient feel better about herself and awaken her sexual longings. The patient was aware of feeling awkward and self-conscious, yet also pleased about the special place she had in her analyst's life. Only years later did she come to recognize how traumatizing these experiences had been.

*Any* theory can be misused in this way. Therapeutic repair can slide into parental and then eroticized touch. Sexual fantasies can be analyzed in a way that itself creates "seductive excess" and slides in the direction of actual seduction.

Our protection against this slide lies in community—in our willingness to see and name these breaches collectively. Yet it's the rare community that has effectively addressed this issue with its members, much less with the larger psychoanalytic world. While violators are sometimes forced to leave their institute, most often they reestablish themselves elsewhere. Their leave-takings tend to be kept quiet; facts remain scarce.

## Is this merely gossip?

When sexual boundary violations at one of my institutes came to light, intense gossip *and* public silence dominated. In part, this was because the administration was legally constrained: Attorneys insisted on complete discretion. Unavoidable though these constraints may be, they mystify—indeed gaslight—the wider professional community and particularly candidates in training.

Often all that's left is whispered gossip. We find an Other, or a few others, with whom to share what we suspect or know. Gossip allows us to remain above the fray while enjoying the charge of an erotically colored shocking story. But rather than serving as an emotional envelope within which to contain, process, and work through disturbing feelings, gossip intensifies our anxiety and distress. It leaves us disrupted rather than relieved; it provides no opportunity for emotional exploration or working through.

The Hebrew equivalent of gossip is *lashon hara* (evil speech), a term that captures the very charged bad feelings—and intent—that this kind of gossip embodies. We become disrupted rather than relieved. To make matters worse, this transgressive element becomes part of our professional legacy, lodged in a kind of psychoanalytic collective unconscious.

Gossip takes place almost exclusively between friends or in very small groups. Indeed, when two sexual violations—one old and one current—came up in a class of 10 that I taught, we all avoided naming the violating faculty members. Several people declared that it would be libelous to do so (even though we all knew whom we were talking about and that these were facts, not rumors). The conversation turned instead to a transgressor from a different institute whose story had been publicized in the press. It was safe to name him; he was "other," neither personally beloved (idealized) nor powerful in our institute. When it comes to our own, we remain mute[2].

Our silence may appear to protect our community, but it doesn't. If anything, it supports a kind of group illusion/delusion that makes it near impossible for us as individuals—and institutions—to contain or metabolize violations without doing major damage to our professional self-image and group identity. To our family.

And paradoxically, even as I try to surface this dynamic here, I also enact it: I describe very disturbing events but don't name the institutes I'm referring to or the transgressors about whom I'm speaking. I leave you, the reader, guessing. Do I mystify more than clarify? Do I arouse curiosity and anxiety, thereby perpetuating the very issue I'm trying to unpack? Do I inadvertently create yet more silent, silenced witnesses?

I'm tempted to name a name, to actively break into this collusion. It would have to be the name of someone deceased or someone already identified in the press, someone who couldn't sue me or my institute.

2  Describing her own experience as a patient, Dimen (2011) addressed the forces silencing patient, analyst, and institute. She, like me, refrained from naming the violator.

On one level, doing so would be relieving. But on another level, I'd feel more disturbed than relieved. Naming the perpetrator could have a destructive impact on his former patients, colleagues, and students, those he didn't abuse. What would be gained by naming someone who's no longer a danger to his patients? It's those I *cannot* name who remain a danger; it's the perpetrators who are alive and active I'm really worried about. And even here, naming names is problematic. In the process of identifying some, I'd be leaving others out, creating some scapegoats while inadvertently protecting other transgressors. There seems to be no exit.

There's something else to consider: How will you—the reader—experience all this? What if you yourself were victim or witness to a sexual violation? What if I break into your disavowal—if it's *your* analyst, colleague, or friend who was, or is, a violator or victim? Will you feel anger at the violator for breaching your trust? Exposure as your secret is partially unmasked? Guilt because you remained silent? Shame over not reporting your abuse or the abuse you witnessed? Jealousy and hurt (over *not* having been chosen as a "special" patient or confidant)? And if you were/are "only" a witness, how upset *are* you entitled to feel? After all, it didn't happen to you.

When first working on this essay, I naïvely assumed I'd be addressing a readership of bystanders and witnesses—those who dwelled outside the arena of actual violations. Only later did it dawn on me that some readers might have (or might be currently) committing a boundary violation. Will this chapter open reflective space, make room for you to own and explore the dynamics behind what you did or are doing? Or will it invite disavowal?

Disavowal is a formidable defense, one that reflects the magnitude of the traumatic disturbance it sidelines. And I know this from the inside because I encountered my own disavowal while writing this essay: About 25 years after I finished my first analysis, I learned that my former analyst had left her husband for a patient. My ex-analyst and I were sometimes in touch, and I (naïvely) communicated my distress to her. Unsurprisingly, she became extremely angry and defensive. The interaction was difficult and disappointing, but it was what happened next that represented a major boundary breach.

A few days later I received a long and hostile phone message from my ex-analyst's partner (whom I didn't know). She not only defended my former analyst but made clear she knew quite a lot about me and used that knowledge to attack me personally. Her viciousness left me shaken. Clearly, my ex-analyst had shared personal information about me with her partner. Her partner's retaliatory, threatening phone call evoked a mixture of hurt, outrage, and vulnerability as I tried to digest the fact my analyst had betrayed my trust.

Probably because this treatment relationship was decades old and I had come to see my former analyst in a shaded rather than idealized way, I was less upset with her than I might have been. Still, it's astonishing to me that, until I wrote this essay, I hadn't realized that a second boundary violation had been committed—against me. My analyst betrayed her patient-lover first, but she also betrayed me, along with her other patients and ex-patients. She upended my professional ideal twice by breaching sexual boundaries with her own patient and then by failing to honor the privileged nature of our relationship. I had managed to sideline the fact that I had been both witness *and* victim. How difficult to metabolize, even 30 years out!

I spoke to a colleague who knew us both; he, while responding supportively and condemning her behavior, didn't call it a boundary breach. Neither of us even considered reporting what had happened! Over time, I "forgot" all about it, forgot so completely that I wrote my first paper on this topic without awareness that I wrote as both witness and as victim.

Former patients who learn of, but are not the victim of, boundary violations are in a position like that of a non-abused child whose sibling is being abused. While there's often no emotional choice except to keep the secret, the peripheral traumatic element is assimilated on a procedural level where it festers and disturbs.

I'm suggesting that we fail to contain violations because we're invested in them. But in mystifying what's known, we confront a different danger— the feeling that we're complicit, that we are, in part, collaborators, both as individuals and as a professional community. At bottom, our very complex feelings about boundary violations reflect a powerful, mostly unconscious need to retain an exalted analytic ideal. That exalted ideal precludes doubleness and thus is vulnerable to shatter.

## A wistful wish

If we're to move beyond this impasse, we need to encompass the possibility that truly reprehensible professional behavior can coexist with a capacity for good analytic work and intellectual brilliance. Is it possible for us to open a space within which to do this?

Could we create our own version of the South African Truth and Reconciliation Commission (M. Moskowitz, personal communication, April 17, 2013)? There, the victims of unspeakable violence confronted their abusers. The possibility of restorative justice was created when harm was fully acknowledged, and in some instances, amnesty from prosecution was given[3].

Might our professional communities create a similar kind of restorative justice system for both the victims and perpetrators of boundary violations? This would mean approaching our colleagues directly but privately when we think they might have committed or might be committing boundary violations. And doing the same with those we suspect are victims.

The victims of major boundary violations write about their experiences in essays and books (e.g., Deutsch, 2014; Dimen, 2011), while protecting the violator's name and the setting in which the breach occurred. This is a first step toward the kind of restorative process I'm thinking about. But it doesn't go nearly far enough; we need to create a safe space in which such a process can happen publicly. A space in which perpetrators acknowledge what happened as a first step toward rehabilitation. Where victim and perpetrator speak to each other directly. Where state law and local governing associations such as the American Psychological Association grant amnesty from criminal prosecution in instances where full disclosure, remorse, and reparation occur. Can we even fathom such a process separate from legal action and banishment?

I'm not sure. But to even contemplate doing this, we need to acknowledge what we know. Aloud. To speak. Together. This means accepting that some of our exalted analytic heroes were—and are—also violators. With the fact that we who would *never* breach a sexual boundary nevertheless commit small but disturbing analytic infractions.

We psychoanalysts have much to be proud about—and much to be ashamed of. How ironic that we who embrace the clinical value of paradox and emotional complexity have so much difficulty encompassing

---

3 Beginning in 1995, the South African Truth and Reconciliation Commission invited victims to publicly describe their experience. Perpetrators could petition for amnesty from prosecution in return for acknowledging their actions. Amnesty was granted to those who told the "whole truth" and whose crimes were "politically motivated" (of course, these are subjective assessments).

what threatens to disrupt our psychoanalytic ideals. We're too often pulled to negate the nonideal because the threat of traumatic de-idealization is unbearable.

If we're to confront our silence and its dynamics, if we're to address the experience of victims, perpetrators, and witnesses and attempt repair, we need to speak together about what we know, feel, and are afraid to say. We need to revisit our relationship to our personal and professional ideals and make peace with the limitations of this profession. Honig and Barron (2013) give us a model to follow in their description of an institute's responses to a sexual boundary violation. Barbara Pizer (2000) proposes that we require ongoing consultation across our analytic lifetime as a wedge against them.

I very much doubt we'll ever succeed in putting a full stop on sexual—or nonsexual—boundary violations, but we might find ways to address their impact on the professional community and our participation in them were we less wedded to a rigid vision of the field and ourselves. It is time, isn't it?

# Chapter 8

# Sequels

Psychoanalytic sequels—post-termination friendships between analyst and patient—are an open secret. Though hardly uncommon, sequels are rarely mentioned, much less explored. Using the unfinished story of a good treatment and its yet-to-be-defined ending to illustrate, I interrogate the complexities of treatment sequels for both patient and analyst.

Sarah began a second analysis with me about a decade ago. Despite a good marriage and satisfying clinical career, her life had been marred by a volatile family relationship that ultimately fractured. Sarah carried the hurt and loss of that fracture across time; it colored and marred the present. And it was another fracture that brought her to me for analysis: Her first analyst, while initially helpful, became rejecting in ways that evoked that early trauma. Distressed and bereft, Sarah wanted help dealing with her failed treatment, its early resonances, and another problematic relationship.

Reflective and insightful, Sarah addressed her failed treatment and its historical antecedents. As we identified her contribution to the analytic impasse and the reenactment it embodied, Sarah began to extricate herself from several troublesome social and collegial involvements. She partly repaired the family rupture that had so plagued her and formed some cleaner and more satisfying professional connections.

Sarah's relationships—inner and actual—deepened and steadied. Moving beyond hurt and anger, she now mostly lived in her very good present.

I thus wasn't surprised when Sarah began to talk about termination. No longer feeling chronically rejected or driven by an urgent need to rework old ties, she wanted time and money to pursue other interests. This seemed right to me too, and we set a termination date about six months ahead. That period together felt rich, a bit sad, but also joyful. After all, it's rare that an analytic couple end treatment feeling satisfied with where it lands.

DOI: 10.4324/9781032691534-12

But here's the rub: Sarah didn't want to say a final goodbye. With tact and hesitancy, she broached the question: She knew it wasn't traditional, but she wondered whether I'd be willing to consider maintaining a connection after termination. Could we allow a collegial relationship to grow, develop into a friendship? We were in the same profession, after all; our overlaps would make this seem almost natural. What, if anything, would I be comfortable with?

Sarah had never pushed treatment boundaries. Yet our many overlaps made me less taken aback by her request than I might have been. Sarah and I share a lot that goes beyond psychoanalysis: we like the same music and films; we're involved in similar political causes; we're both Jewishly identified. Over the years we'd bumped into each other at both psychoanalytic and nonprofessional events (yes, Manhattan is a village); those chance encounters had felt warm and easy. I thus wasn't altogether surprised by Sarah's request, despite its collision both with analytic norms and Sarah's bounded way of being. Reacting with a simultaneous sense of pleasure at her request and caution about breaching a boundary I had held to firmly over decades, I hesitated. How to respond?

I use this vignette to introduce the theme of analytic desire as it informs, enriches, and traumatically disrupts psychoanalytic endings and transformations. For despite the place of honor we've accorded termination, both need and desire—analyst's as well as the patient's—shape the ways we end and the ways we don't.

I begin by delineating the borders of the question I raise. I'm *not* addressing post-analytic sexual relationships or other kinds of boundary crossings involving sexual, financial, or other deliberate exploitation of the patient. The danger of "coasting in the countertransference" (Hirsch, 2008) is ubiquitous. But deliberately using a patient to satisfy one's own needs, of enacting personal desire or greed, irreparably harms the patient and the treatment; there's a clear line in the sand that precludes such engagements.

Of course, that line is regularly breached (chapters 6 and 7). Serious boundary crossings take many forms, the most common (and perhaps most problematic) being sexual violations (Alpert & Steinberg, 2017; Celenza, 2007, 2017, 2021; Crown, 2017; Dimen, 2011; Gabbard, 1995a, 1995b; Gabbard & Lester, 1995; Goren, 2017; Grossmark, 2017; Slochower, 2017b, 2017c). Our profession is deeply disturbed by these phenomena, but neither dynamic exploration nor legal action has disrupted their prevalence. How can we expect that less flagrant boundary crossings would even break the surface of our inattention?

Nonsexual post-treatment relationships have been part of our professional lives since our earliest beginnings (Bergmann, 1988). Indeed, analysts have virtually institutionalized ways of sustaining relationships with ex-analysands across the lifetime (Pedder, 1988; Wallerstein, 1986). Post-analytic connections are written into the structure of institute life and create ongoing occasions for contact. We see each other at meetings, parties, and professional gatherings. We work together in a variety of contexts. Most candidates anticipate this (Levine & Yanof, 2004; Schachter, 1992). It's difficult to know just how this affects the treatment experience for candidate analysands and their analysts, but it certainly must.

Post-treatment friendships are less common when the patient isn't in the field, but they're not unheard of. A range of non-psychoanalytic overlaps (concrete and not) can open the door to a post-treatment connection (more about this shortly). It's nevertheless more typical for termination with a non-analyst patient to end all contact between the two unless the patient seeks the analyst out for more analysis.

How ironic that we ask of our non-analyst patients something most of us are never called on to do: Face the starkness of a complete ending (Pedder, 1988)!

## Why terminate?

Because termination has its own therapeutic impact (Bergmann, 1988, 1997; Frankiel, 2007; Freud, 1914; Pedder, 1988; Slochower, 1998a). Salberg (2009, 2010) invites us to think and theorize about when, how, and why we terminate. Kantrowitz (2015) explores the vicissitudes of termination and their impact on analyst and patient from the analyst patient's point of view.

A good termination goes like this: Patient and analyst set a mutually agreed-upon end date, work toward it, and end. And for good reason: Good-enough endings deepen and expand analytic work. Indeed, Renik (1991, 1996, 1999) suggests that defining a termination date may itself be a necessary condition for analytic progress. Life-and-death anxieties (Coltart, 1996) are evoked, separation issues stimulated, old object ties rekindled. Working through all this will facilitate the resolution of themes including (though not limited to) relinquishment and internalization. Gradually, the transference is resolved, the analytic relationship decathected, and identification with the analyst takes its place (Frankiel, 2007; Loewald, 1960; Weinshel & Renik, 1991). The analyst is absorbed as a steady presence and remembered; in the process, an inner tie is integrated and a capacity for self-analysis consolidated (Loewald, 1988; Schachter, 1992; Tessman, 2003). Increasingly, the patient is freed psychically and relationally; self-analytic functions develop, releasing the patient from dependence on the analyst's analyzing capacity and facilitating a move toward separateness. Part of a successful termination process will involve analysts' engagement with their own countertransference.

Yet most of us know that "complete terminations" are rare. Schachter (1992) notes that only about half of analytic patients reach a mutually agreed-upon endpoint. Levine and Yanof (2004) and Yanof and Levine (2005) conducted an informal study of post-analytic contact between ex-analysands and their analysts. Although they underscore its problematic implications, they also argue that post-analytic contact should be individually evaluated and isn't inherently a boundary violation.

But failing to fully terminate—let alone developing a friendship or other kind of relationship with a former patient—collides with our analytic ideal; specifically, with our termination ideal. After all, analysis is supposed to help people move on in *their* lives, not in ours. Continuing the treatment tie post-termination runs the risk of enacting, rather than working through, the residual transference element and the wishes it embodies.

Such enactments can subvert the ex-patient's emotional investment in other relationships and keep the patient tied to the analyst in unanalyzable ways. Like other boundary violations, they can simultaneously exploit and obfuscate the patient's underlying need—for example, for a parental connection. Even when this isn't the case, the extension of the analysis into the social realm interferes with optimal disillusionment; it will likely truncate, if not foreclose, mourning processes and the working through they can facilitate.

## Crossing the analytic line

Like many smaller professional delinquencies, establishing a nonsexual relationship after termination raises eyebrows but usually not much more. In part, that's because we rarely know enough to ascertain, much less pass judgment on, what has happened or is happening. We don't know what informed the analyst's decision to agree to (or instigate) a post-treatment relationship, or what the particulars of that relationship are. We cannot assess its impact on the patient. Further, both the analyst's and patient's conscious understandings and motives will likely mask the underlying emotional complexities of such a move.

On an interpersonal level, turning a circumscribed, transference-based relationship into a "real" relationship crosses a challenging line. The asymmetry characteristic of the treatment setup (Aron, 1991) may remain a shadow presence that colors, even skews, the "newly" constructed friendship. An overtly platonic friendship could, for example, obscure an underlying sexual element. Alternatively, the treatment's therapeutic dimension may be carried forward into the friendship so that the patient continues to "be" a patient—to rely on the ex-analyst for symbolic parental support, advice, even interpretations, albeit over coffee or a meal. At other times this dynamic reverses so that the analyst turns to the patient for help or support. Either way, idealization—asymmetrical or shared—probably remains a shadow presence.

Unpacking the process by which the dyad decides to move from a professional to a personal relationship might clarify its dynamics and ethics. But it's difficult—probably impossible—to do so from the outside. Was the choice to move beyond the professional considered, discussed, and carefully analyzed? Was it made collaboratively or shaped by a residual power differential that left the choice in the hands of one member of the dyad? To the degree that the decision was driven by the wish or need of one party and acquiesced to by the other, we're in the realm of something more potentially coercive than genuinely mutual.

## More than a post-analytic friendship

Not infrequently, post-treatment contact between analyst and patient becomes something more. Ex-analysts sometimes offer—and/or the patient seeks—a kind of mentorship that results in the ex-patient becoming the analyst's protégé. Senior analysts provide all kinds of professional support to their junior colleagues, among them their ex-patients. Especially when the ex-analyst has professional gravitas, that sponsorship can have significant effects, both dynamic and concrete. The ex-analyst may help open professional doors, connect a former patient to powerful colleagues, editors, conference organizers, and so on; beyond the concrete help given, these "gifts" can carry powerful symbolic meaning. Yet they are rarely acknowledged explicitly, let alone analyzed. The original therapeutic relationship tends to go publicly (and often privately) unmentioned, though it may be recognized by some.

More than post-analytic friendships, we take sponsorship connections for granted; indeed, they've become a professional tradition, a way of "passing the baton." But a great deal is at stake dynamically when the ex-patient's sponsor was the analyst. Ex-patients may, for example, feel validated, even buoyed, by their ex-analyst's faith in them. That faith, whether symbolic or enacted, can have a generative impact. Similarly, the analyst may experience both pleasure and a sense of professional power in helping advance the career of an ex-patient.

This kind of sponsorship has an underbelly. It can perpetuate an unspoken interdependence in which the patient continues to rely on the analyst—now for professional advancement—while the analyst derives pleasure from, and may come to rely on, the patient's idealization. Sponsorship relationships can subtly undermine an ex-patient's sense of agency and competence, leaving the erstwhile patient psychologically (if not literally) dependent on the analyst's help. The analyst, now valued for their instrumental power, may inadvertently communicate that the patient cannot—or should not—step beyond the analytic relationship and act independently (theoretically, clinically, or personally). The patient may feel pressured to remain loyal to the analyst and/or to the analyst's point of view. Will the patient whose career flourishes because of this help feel secretly or unconsciously fraudulent, the recipient of nepotism that undercuts a sense of agency and pride in her professional accomplishments? Will it intensify the patient's dependence on the ex-analyst? And what about the analyst? Will underlying guilt or anxiety about what goes unnamed color the analyst's feelings about both members of the dyad? Will the analyst—perhaps unconsciously—feel sullied, even corrupted, in the process?

An equally important aspect of this phenomenon is its impact on the professional community. Like sexual boundary violations that are widely known to have occurred but are never mentioned, protégé relationships remain an open secret. We "know" that X was a patient of Y's and rose to a position of power by riding on the ex-analyst's coattails. But there's no arena in which to acknowledge, let alone explore, this fact or its impact.

Protégé relationships provoke a range of reactions, both in those patients who were not "chosen" and in the wider community. Some judge the dyad; some condemn the analyst, the patient, or both. Some envy the ex-patient's special place with the analyst, feel bitterness about having been passed over, long to be the chosen one. And, like those aware of sexual boundary crossings in the institute community, the larger community may carry a peripheral sense that it is corrupt—that an ethical line has been crossed.

## Our analytic ideal and analytic actuality

The termination ideal is organized around the sanctity of analytic space and its firm borders. Once we end, we're supposed to keep memories but not much more. Perhaps a holiday card, a birth announcement, a return office visit to address a new issue, but not ongoing contact and certainly not social contact (see, e.g., Bonovitz, 2007; Hoffman, 1998; Mitchell, 1993; Witenberg, 1976). I share this view: My own training left me convinced that such liaisons are inherently out of bounds; that we should protect the treatment relationship and remain available to our patient across our lifetime; that a complete termination is a "fence"—an essential protection against the dissolution or corruption of psychoanalytic process and of the analyst.

Ironically, our analytic ideal has had a paradoxical effect on our capacity to acknowledge, let alone explore, the nature, meanings, and complexities of nonsexual post-treatment liaisons (cf., Firestein, 1982; Kantrowitz, 2015). We've mostly evaded thinking, let alone writing, about them. Although many believe that these relationships are transgressive, we're often unsure *how* transgressive they are. And unless sex is involved, we don't even gossip much.

Yet most treatment endings don't quite meet our ideal. Truncated treatments and abrupt endings; terminations avoided, postponed, or refused; patients who resist stopping even when they feel the treatment has been successful and that they're largely "done." Some ask the obvious: Why end when it's so good? Martin Bergmann (1997) noted, "there are analysands for whom transference love, in spite of its lack of physical intimacy, is the best love relationship they ever had" (p. 169). Why should anyone want to give that up?

The power of the analytic connection is sometimes so strong that both patient and analyst respond to the prospect of losing it by convincing themselves there's no need to end, that there's still more work to be done. I've joked (or half-joked) with a few of my patients who declare they'll never terminate by musing aloud about future sessions in which I hobble out to the waiting room and our walkers collide. Not infrequently, we work long and hard on ending and ultimately it happens: A leave-taking that feels good, integrative, strengthening to us both. But not always.

## What the analyst wants

Some decades ago, a colleague lent me a copy of an article on termination that included a statement about how our bonds to our patients are based on our professional function rather than on need. In the margin she wrote "ho ho ho" (Diane Friedman, personal communication, 2012).

I couldn't say it better. We analysts can be just as invested in continuing relationships with our patients as they are—even more invested. If we maintain relationships with patients after termination, we may assert that it's because they, not we, need it. But this may be a rationalized explanation that skips over how inextricably our own wants and needs can be implicated in these decisions. Because analytic self-interest, along with analytic desire, regularly infiltrate therapeutic space and shape what we do and how we rationalize it.

Analysts have their own need to believe that things have been resolved and that the transference relationship has been transformed. We go along with what's pleasurable for our own reasons while sidelining our doubts, no matter superego prohibitions. Wilson (2003, 2020) describes the powerful impact of the analyst's desire—for a particular analytic experience, for a sense of aliveness, for the fulfillment of fantasies, for gratifying contact with the patient. These self-interested desires may include a wish to extend the analytic relationship beyond its border. Might they also invite a mutual resistance to the final analytic ending?[1]

Viorst (1986) details the painful ways in which ending can be experienced by the analyst. When loss feels unbearable, continuing the relationship post-termination can represent a reprieve, even an emotional solution. At other times, it's our sense of disappointment, lack, or grief about the analysis itself that leads us to prolong a treatment relationship. Our conviction that there's more to repair is fueled by our resistance to letting go. We may allow those desires to develop into something else because we,

---

1 Self-interest can also inform the analyst's desire for a complete termination. For example, those who enjoy being idealized may not *want* to be known outside their analytic role; that preference may inform what looks like a clinical decision.

as much—or more—than our patients, want/need that "something more," whether support, admiration, or concrete help.

Protected from the vicissitudes of ordinary love relationships, a post-treatment friendship seems to offer the analyst the kind of idealized loving relationship that cannot exist outside it. For the analyst whose personal relationships are disappointing, conflicted, or absent, the treatment connection may evoke a deep longing to continue past the point of "appropriate" termination. Kubie (1968) suggests that a post-treatment friendship also "creates an opportunity for the analyst to turn to the patient with his own needs. Unconsciously he feels, I have been the giver. 'Now it's my turn to be given'" (p. 345).

None of this is especially surprising. The intensity, richness, and deep knowing that characterizes an analytic connection isn't something we easily give up. If anything, it's remarkable that we sometimes *do* end completely.

When I presented this paper at institutes in the United States and abroad, I always asked if any attendees knew firsthand of nonsexual post-analytic friendships. In every group, at least half a dozen people raised their hands. These friendship connections were either discovered accidentally or because the ex-patient was a close friend who confided in a colleague. In no instance were they "out." This secrecy has made it nearly impossible for us to examine the dynamic impact of these relationships on the analytic couple or on the larger community.

## Revisiting the termination ideal

Our vision of termination reflects, and probably emerges out of, Western developmental perspectives that privilege separation-individuation over attachment and dependence (e.g., Mahler, 1968; Schachter, 1992). To analogize, a focus on the patient's need to separate and develop a sense of autonomy and agency minimizes, even skips over, the value of sustained attachment (S. Stern, 2020). It's thus unsurprising that there's a relative dearth of literature on post-termination contact, let alone post-termination relationships.

Schachter (1992, 2005) and Kantrowitz (2015) are exceptions. Schachter's focus is on planned follow-up analytic contact, not post-treatment friendships. He concludes there's little clinical evidence that post-termination contacts are harmful to the patient. Kantrowitz interviewed 82 ex-analysands about termination. Among the many areas she explores is patients' experience of post-analytic contact. Kantrowitz believes that no generalization can be made because peoples' responses to post-treatment contact are so variable.

For many of our patients, reliable attachment remains an analytic goal more than a given. This is particularly true when early relational trauma interferes with a capacity to develop secure attachments. Here, a complete termination may be both an *après coup* and a new trauma. Traumatized patients may need a softer kind of ending, punctuated rather than absolute, with periodic check-ins or return visits, brief or extended.

We've yet to address this theme outside the arena of trauma. Yet as we move beyond our early emphasis on separation-individuation and reframe our understanding of these developmental processes, we open the door to a more complex perspective on endings. If a capacity for deep attachment—rather than separation per se—is a sign of maturity that needn't reflect undifferentiated merger, complete endings no longer seem the single "right" way to go (see, e.g., Bonovitz, 2007; Davies, 2005; Grand, 2009; Layton, 2010).

In their best iteration, our attachments enrich life while leaving us free to go our own way. Might the treatment relationship sometimes mirror this configuration? Could the analyst-patient dyad develop a post-termination relationship indicative not of unresolved transference issues but rather a move beyond the transference? Might some post-analytic friendships reflect growth and maturity (rather than residual need)? Might both patient and analyst sometimes have the capacity to move past the transference relationship?

Transference-based fantasies don't always simply get worked through and resolved; they sometimes transform in ways that reflect not gratification but personal (and dyadic) maturity. Just as some adult children become friends to their parents and leave dependence behind, some ex-dyads may develop a relationship beyond the reenacted (transference) element, a relationship that's genuinely mutual and egalitarian.

I think of Paul, a former patient who for years reacted with great intensity and distress to any evidence of my separateness. The announcement of an upcoming vacation, for example, would provoke anger and hurt, a feeling that I don't care and/or will forget about him. It took years, but the day arrived when, anticipating this reaction, I said something about knowing how hard my vacations were for him. Paul looked amused and said,

You're stuck in an earlier version of who I was, not who I am. You need to update your file. I'm not there now—I got over that and I now know we're connected. I take it for granted. So I can wish you a good vacation and mean it. As my shrink friends would say, I've become securely attached.

Paul's deepened capacity for mutual relatedness represented an emotional sea change that left him (and me) delighted. The transference element (in which I was mostly experienced as cold and rejecting) had first attenuated and then transformed. We now had a mutual, respectful, and loving connection that lacked the sticky charge dominating much of the analysis.

Paul and I terminated about a year later. He mourned our parting but was also eager to move on in his life. He never raised the question of continuing our connection and I never contemplated our becoming friends. As I write this paper, though, I retrospectively wonder whether, had we made such a move, it might have embodied the transformation of our connection from one embedded in transference-based need toward one mutually enriching and gratifying.

Or is this going too far? *Can* the transference so fully resolve that the patient will leave behind the longings, conflicts, and anxieties it evokes? Can the ex-patient experience the analyst as a new object without the transference element? What about patients' need to mourn the loss of the analyst as a valuable emotional process in its own right? These two themes—the need to mourn and work through loss *and* to sustain attachments across time—are, after all, both central analytic goals.

Certainly, the truism "once a patient, always a patient" underscores both the value of termination and the risks associated with not terminating. Won't residues of idealized love (and hate) inevitably remain, a consequence of transference's intensity? Reich (1958), Pfeffer (1963), Kubie (1968), Loewald (1988), and Bergmann (1988) all believe that elements of the transference persist after the end of the analysis. From this perspective, a "complete" working through of the transference happens seldom, if ever. And even if this is occasionally not the case, how can we differentiate a genuinely mutual friendship from a problematic one?

It's easy enough to find illustrations of this kind of problematic reversal. Some years after completing her analysis, a colleague and her former analyst found themselves at the same vacation spot quite by chance. My colleague told me about it:

> I was delighted to see her, and she seemed pleased to see me too. We had a lot of catching up to do and it felt really equal and warm. Then an airline strike left us both stranded and I discovered that I am much more practically competent than she. She didn't know what to do; I helped her rebook her flight and so on—she was flummoxed. Not a big deal, but it set the stage for a kind of reversal because now whenever we speak, she asks me for help with something concrete. On one hand I like this role; I'm needed and that feels good. On the other hand, I'm aware that it's got a downside; I don't always *want* to be the helper and it's also kind of undone my sense of my ex-analyst's competence.

My colleague illustrates what Bergmann (1988) noted: That a "real" relationship with an ex-analyst can disappoint more than please. Only when the treatment relationship moved beyond the consulting room did what originally seemed so special become sufficiently upended to leave the former patient disappointed and somewhat disillusioned. The de-idealization my colleague describes might be thought of as a realistic reassessment, as emerging in the space between the ideal and the actual *or* as evidence that the post-analytic friendship contained a significant residual transference element that hadn't been worked through.

In principle, the decision to become friends after treatment should be mutual. But the asymmetry characteristic of the analytic situation may obfuscate what underlies this: Namely, that despite appearances to the contrary, this decision ultimately rests in the analyst's hands *even if the patient initiates this shift*. In this sense, the analytic past remains a ghostly absence/presence lurking in or beneath these conversations (Kalb, 2021). If that ghost can be named, unpacked, and talked about, a genuine transformation that includes the residue of the early asymmetry may take place. But we cannot exclude the possibility that an "as if" accommodation obscures the patient's compliance with the analyst's needs and desires.

Further complicating matters is the fact that post-treatment connections remain a partially public secret. Might that secrecy allow the analyst to commit other kinds of delinquencies? That is, do post-treatment friendships invite a slide down the slope toward problematic boundary violations?

And there are other risks. A colleague who became friends with an ex-patient told me he had discovered he didn't much like who the patient was as a person. In "real" life, he found the patient rather self-centered and awkward. Not having viewed the patient this way in treatment, my colleague felt disillusioned. He also felt caught, unable to say anything about what he felt, to exit the friendship, or address what had changed.

Idealization, de-idealization, as-ifness, exploitation, rupture, and a sense of obligation all threaten to color, if not spoil, a post-analytic relationship. Yet despite our belief that these relationships are out of bounds, analysts sometimes do become—and remain—friends with former patients in ways that feel valuable to both parties. My colleague Andrew described this evolution:

> We've been bumping into each other at professional meetings for years. We kept a distance initially, but over time it gave way to a warm connection. I feel easy with him and he seems to feel easy as well. I certainly don't idealize him; there are things about him that I find annoying and I'm sure that's true for him, too. I remain grateful for his analytic help and am pleased that I've had the privilege of sustaining that relationship beyond the end of the treatment. There's a warm, easy kind of mutual knowing between us that reflects the depth of the work we did together, I think.
>
> What's odd, given what I know about transference, is that I can't find any residue of it between us anymore. You may be skeptical; I was, too, for a long time. I recognize that this may be defensive, but I actually don't think it is. I can't find a way in which this friendship has been harmful to me. It didn't preclude other relationships or leave me stuck. It has enriched my life, and I think his as well.

Of course, we needn't take Andrew's words at face value. Transference feelings and fantasies lurk at the edges of nearly all our relationships—how can Andrew be so sure that his don't? Might he not be unconsciously invested in denying or disavowing the complexities coloring his experience with his former analyst? And, though I cannot interview his analyst, must not he, too, have needs that are implicated here?

Still. An open and self-reflective person, Andrew articulates the other side of the termination ideal. He feels enriched by his connection with his former analyst; he consciously experiences neither guilt nor conflict about it. Rather than its having had a problematic impact on his life or other connections, Andrew feels that this post-termination friendship is a marker of his emotional transformation. Can we trust this? Or is there more there than meets the eye?

## When the patient isn't an analyst

Post-termination connections most frequently emerge out of professional overlaps. Or at least, friendships between ex-patient and ex-analyst are more evident to us. When the patient isn't in the field, post-treatment connections easily remain hidden from view. It's difficult to obtain data on their frequency or assess their impact on analyst and patient, but they do occur.

I think of an ex-patient and ex-analyst who both love an unusual kind of music. They often bumped into each other at concerts; over the years they became friends. That friendship's secrecy is easy to sustain; few know about the dyad's clinical past.

Still other post-treatment friendships coalesce not out of concrete overlaps but because of a more ephemeral—but equally powerful—personal bond that creates a sense of being kindred spirits. Unfortunately, as Kantrowitz (2015) notes, there are no studies of these post-treatment liaisons that would allow us to evaluate their frequency or psychological impact.

## Open and shut: Our failure to ritualize

Despite the joy, sense of accomplishment, and freedom that accompany a successful termination, ending is a loss for both patient and analyst. The belief that all the necessary mourning can take place during the termination period itself leaves both parties quite alone once final goodbyes are said.

Our psychoanalytic perspective on termination mirrors early models of mourning. Both actual death and the end of an analysis are bounded processes with emotional endpoints and clear goals. The lost object is internalized, freeing the person to move forward. Only insecure, ambivalent attachment or the dynamics associated with pathological mourning were believed to interfere with resolution (Akhtar & Smolar, 1998; Bergmann, 1997). The need for ongoing acts of mourning was viewed as evidence of underlying early trauma. "Ordinary" loss is resolved via internalization of the absent object (Bassin, 1998; Bernstein, 2000; Volkan, 2007).

But wait. Doesn't significant loss—not only traumatic loss—require ongoing acts of remembrance? Commemorative ritual—personal, cultural, or religious—emerges out of our need to mark and periodically evoke our losses across the lifespan, whether or not those losses were traumatic (Slochower, 2015a). From this perspective, it's not clear that the termination process alone can provide sufficient opportunity to mourn, remember, and grieve the ending of what is, for some, the most intimate and rich relationship of their lives.

Freud himself came to recognize that profound mourning isn't easily resolved. In 1929 he wrote a personal letter to his friend Ludwig Binswanger, offering condolences on the death of Binswanger's son. (It seems likely that Freud was also articulating his own grief over the death of his daughter Sophie, who died of the Spanish flu, and his grandson Heinerle, who died of tuberculosis)[2].

> Although . . . the acute state of mourning will subside . . . we shall remain inconsolable and will never find a substitute. No matter what may fill the gap, even if it be filled completely, it nevertheless remains something else. And actually, this is how it should be. It is the only way of perpetuating that love which we do not want to relinquish.
>
> (Freud, 1929)

Here, Freud identifies something I would apply to the analytic situation itself: Acute feelings of loss may be carried across time, long beyond the initial mourning process.

Mourning the loss of the analytic relationship is, at least at times, a far less circumscribed process than was originally thought (Buechler, 2000; Cooper, 2000; Craige, 2002, 2006). I say this even though there's also much potential gain in the termination process. When an analytic ending is jointly arrived at, rather than unilaterally chosen or imposed by external factors, grief at saying goodbye may be mitigated, even overridden, by a sense of exhilaration, joy, by a shared recognition of all that's been accomplished. Patient and analyst have an opportunity to celebrate what has changed, to work through the ending together before actual goodbyes are said.

---

2 On another level, he may also have been alluding to the loss of his symbolic son (Ferenczi) and his conflict with Jones (Steve Ellman, personal communication, 2022).

Still, termination is stark: The final analytic goodbye closes off access to the only "like mourner"—the only "other" who shared the relationship that has now ended. Ironically, this analytic other is both alive and absent—unreachable as a partner or as a witness to a longer commemorative process.

The end of an analysis, then, leaves us without opportunities for remembrance: There's no anniversary to mark, no symbolic or literal grave to visit, no shared rituals of remembrance, culturally or religiously embedded affective symbols, container for loss or absence, and no holding space (Bassin, 2003). Both patient and analyst are now alone with a loss that's difficult to commemorate with anyone other than the lost other. I think this can be true even though loss is only one of many feelings that follow a good termination.

## What the analyst loses

Our termination ideal occludes the relational void that follows the end of an analysis. That void isn't altogether dissimilar from what can be felt following other life markers (e.g., graduation, retirement, a move to another state or country); all tend to evoke a sense of both exhilaration and sadness. But it's mainly in analysis that we lack the opportunity to share the experience of loss with "like" mourners over time. Only here is there a prohibition against refinding the "lost" (but still alive) other. Calling an ex-analyst (or ex-patient) to say we miss them, that we want to catch up, would typically raise eyebrows, be read as a sign of unfinished analytic work. Equally eyebrow-raising would be our affirmative response to such a request from an ex-patient.

Analysts rarely write about their own sense of loss at termination, let alone their wish to continue a relationship with a former patient, but we too can suffer from these absences and longings. No wonder we write essays about our patients, our relationships with them, our own treatment. But while there are many essays in our literature describing the emotional impact of successful and failed analyses, nearly all are written from the patient's perspective. There's a limit to what we can comfortably say about our investment in continuing a connection to our patient post-treatment, or our sadness and loss when someone we've cared deeply about says a final goodbye. Our commitment to helping people move on in their lives collides with our personal grief at losing those we care about.

On one level, establishing a post-analytic friendship solves this problem. When the therapeutic tie is transformed into a personal one, patient and analyst simultaneously evade and enact the commemorative rituals foreclosed by termination. Might some post-treatment friendships be, at least in part, implicit acts of commemorative ritual? Are they, at bottom, an attempt to find our way back to the only "like mourner"—our analytic partner, someone who also witnessed and experienced the end of the analysis?

## What kind of friends are we?

I'm not sure it's possible to fully define a post-analytic relationship; its therapeutic history precludes our calling it either a simple friendship or an extended therapeutic tie. Where the analytic relationship provides the patient a witness, even a scaffolding, that supports new relational and psychic capacities, a post-treatment connection *should* be less tilted toward patient need and more dyadically formulated; at times it may even tilt toward the analyst's need. But no matter how egalitarian, this friendship has a nonegalitarian history that can't be entirely erased.

Can this dynamic evolve over time? Is it possible for analyst and patient to become like subjects (Benjamin, 1995a), no longer embedded in an asymmetrical relationship? And can a post-analytic connection to the ex-analyst represent a marker of therapeutic success rather than failure?

It's undoubtedly safer to say no. But I'm wondering whether there are instances in which we do our patients a disservice by rejecting their wish to continue a connection to us. Could this wish sometimes reflect a new relational capacity that deserves to be honored rather than pathologized?

I want to challenge and complicate the idealization of separation inherent in the termination ideal. That idealization has shadowed us and narrowed our analytic goals by sidestepping the potential value of deep, sustained attachment to the ex-analyst across time. Interestingly, this has been true across theoretical divides; it applies to both classical and relational/interpersonal theories, and to those in between.

Certainly, the capacity for rich, nonconflictual attachments leans on a solid sense of separateness. In the absence of the latter, our connections tend to become adhesive, conflicted, or limiting. We need to first establish ourselves as ourselves before we can freely connect to the other. And patients differ with regard to both capacities. Some need to develop or consolidate a sense of separateness. Here our aim is to facilitate autonomous, steady I-thou relatedness in which the other's experience no longer occludes the patient's own, in which the development and integration of a sense of boundaries dominates (chapters 1 and 2). But for others, it's the need for deep and sustained connectedness that's lacking.

Which brings me back to Sarah. As we addressed the dynamics that derailed her previous treatment, we worked on her experience of what sounded to me like the analyst's withholding, punitive stance. We explored her contribution to the treatment's relative failure and addressed those elements when they emerged (in a quieter form) in our relationship. As we unpacked the reenacted element, we identified and worked on an unconscious pull toward critical, rejecting parental ties.

While initially avoidant of intimacy and hiding need, Sarah had moved toward mature engagement. She developed a wider emotional range despite some continued avoidance of intimacy. Now less sensitive to slights, Sarah's stormy relationships with her adult children quieted. Her marriage, always a good one, deepened and felt more satisfying. Increasingly, she was able to deal with the ordinary. And she had become more (if not altogether) prepared for the unthinkable.

At first, I was wary of stepping into the kind of adhesive transference that had characterized Sarah's earlier treatment. But as time passed and the work deepened, that wariness—in tandem with Sarah's defensiveness—dissipated and transformed into a sense of easy engagement. Sarah was relaxed, open, and nonintrusive, yet warmly related. Might we be capable of transforming the treatment relationship into a mutual one and moving beyond the shadow of what came before?

If there were a patient with whom I could justify extending the treatment tie post-termination because of a trauma history, it would not be Sarah. Although she had some underlying attachment issues, she had mostly moved past them. And Sarah's early life, while difficult in some ways, hadn't seriously derailed her; she grew up a resilient, sturdy child. Over the course of the treatment, her capacity for emotional depth, self-reflectivity, and affect regulation became increasingly stable and solid. Sarah no longer struggled with the transference issues that brought her into treatment. Importantly, our relationship was never especially sticky; although the transference element periodically emerged between us in a quiet form, it mostly remained with her previous analyst.

I use the case of Sarah to illustrate a clinical conundrum many of us have encountered at some point in our practice: The wish to make an exception, to ignore or override the termination ideal just this once. Can we trust our assessment of the role of wish and need (our own and our patient's) in moving toward a post-treatment friendship? Were both my wish (to become friends with Sarah) and denial (of underlying dynamics) implicated here? After all, we analysts are ourselves vulnerable to what Josephs (1995) calls "tunnel vision."

Whether a post-analytic friendship is initiated by the patient or by the analyst, seriously entertaining it threatens to evoke the analytic police, a significant internalized element to be contended with. For most of us, the eleventh commandment is to privilege patient need over our own desire. Not to act on impulse. The only acceptable road to continuing contact with a former patient would lie in that patient's fragility and trauma history, in her need not to lose yet another emotional connection. That perspective, if not simply a rationalization, privileges our patient's need, certainly not our own desire. Would a no to Sarah reflect a rigid or appropriate clinical judgment? And what might be obscured were I to say yes?

In more than 40 years of analytic practice, I've never even considered becoming friends with an ex-patient, even with ex-analysands who were in the field. Yet Sarah's tactfully worded request confronted me with a collision between the ideal and the actual. I felt that collision acutely. After all, I chaired the Division 39 Ethics Committee for nearly a decade. I've written papers on analytic self-interest and on sexual and nonsexual boundary violations. How could I, of all people, even consider doing this?

And why with Sarah? She isn't someone with significant residual trauma, so it's hard for me to justify a move to friendship based on her need. Sarah feels, consciously at least, that she doesn't *need* me in her life; she *wants* me in her life, as a colleague, peer, and friend. She asked if we could meet occasionally for coffee, a walk in the park. The particulars didn't matter— what mattered was sustaining our connection across time. What might I be comfortable with? Sarah wanted the decision to be a joint one.

Though touched by Sarah's recognition of my subjectivity, I held back. I said I wanted to remain available as her analyst. Becoming friends would muddy things, get in the way of a more complete working through. And might there be more to her request than met the eye? Might we still have work to do? If she were set on ending, perhaps we could plan a check-in session later in the year. Sarah replied:

I suspected you'd say something like that. And I can't argue with you since I know that there's always an unconscious level to things. But it's really not what I want. To come here as your patient would feel "as if" to me. It would kind of negate who I've become and what has gone on between us. Of the fact that I've really matured. It's "Joyce the person," not "Joyce the analyst" I want to keep in my life. I know that if we were to become friends, I wouldn't be able to return for further treatment should the need arise. I don't think it will, but if it did, I'd see someone else.

There was something about Sarah's response that felt authentic, mature, and mutual. I felt moved, and my reluctance began to give way to a wish to give it a try.

But. When we encounter our desire to establish a post-treatment friendship, we may not only skip over its dynamic complexity, we may also be unaware of what that relationship would feel like. Residues of the earlier therapeutic bond could result in a feeling of strain and difficulty. The parental (transference) element could leave me feeling awkward, wanting to maintain boundaries with Sarah. To limit how much I self-disclose. All this might coalesce into a frustrating quality of constraint that would feel disappointing to us both. It could leave Sarah (and/or me) feeling unable to rock the relational boat by asking for more or unconsciously pressured to sound psychologically "together." And if our friendship turned out to be difficult for either of us, the fear of hurting the other could leave one or both of us feeling unable to back out of the relationship.

Considering the possibility of becoming friends with a patient also challenges the superego residue of analytic training, whatever its particulars. Does a sense of cynicism or disillusionment with analytic work in an analyst's later years pull us this way? Desire or loneliness? Might aging and the prospect of finite endings be implicated here? Aging tends to pull us analysts away from professional "should"—toward our humanity and away from old rigidities (Chapter 11). Toward a need to mourn and commemorate. And perhaps toward a new vision of analytic endings.

### Complicating our termination ideal: What's at risk?

When we train candidates, we tend to emphasize analytic shoulds and should-nots. Certainly, there's considerable cross-theoretical variability in how we formulate the frame. But whatever the particulars of our ideal, we want our candidates (and colleagues) to adhere to it.

What would the implications of loosening that termination ideal be? If we implicitly invite new candidates to ignore or sidestep it, don't we undermine our sense of professional self-esteem? And what of our other patients, those with whom we do end completely? Would they suffer from feeling less valued/important/loved? We might inadvertently set up a "most favored" analytic subgroup that would generate—or at least intensify—envy and/or competition among candidates.

Beyond the personal, there are risks for the field. Post-termination relationships could invite a new kind of intergenerational transmission that compromises our commitment to the analytic ideal. It could make the profession appear—or become—corrupt, guilty of self-interested boundary breaches. It could create a slide away from core psychoanalytic principles and toward self-indulgence.

Experience and analytic maturity are requisites for making this choice in a responsible, principled way. But experience is no guarantee of maturity. Senior analysts, decades beyond their training and assimilation of analytic rules, may be *more* vulnerable to the invasion of self-interest than their younger colleagues and more pulled toward post-treatment connections. But, of course, professional slippage doesn't reside squarely in the arena of post-termination friendships. Analysts justify, rationalize, or ignore the potential dangers of all kinds of complex or problematic choices. There's no exit from this kind of professional vulnerability.

## Analytic ideals and relational actuality

We analysts aim high, perhaps too high. We require of ourselves a near superhuman capacity to focus on the other and to explore our dynamics as they inform the process.

Our own wants are not supposed to be enacted. But inevitably, they are. And to some extent they shape how we end—and how we don't. We analysts can find ourselves caught between what we believe we shouldn't want and what we need *not* to need. Our needs and our theory, in concert with our patient's wishes and fears, can foreclose awareness of the complex factors that inform the decision both to terminate *and* to continue a relationship post-termination. The pressure of the termination ideal, along with our overactive (or underactive) analytic superego, can foreclose scrutiny of the anti-ideal, the possibility that not ending a relationship when we end an analysis may be enriching for some patients and some analysts some of the time.

Most patients need to end treatment in their own time, to say goodbye and be on their way. They leave full of pleasure as well as sadness. Most analysts need this too.

As Winnicott (1962) noted,

> Having begun an analysis, I expect to continue with it, to survive it and to end it. I enjoy myself doing analysis and I always look forward to the end of each analysis.

(p. 165)

I do think Winnicott overstates a bit here, both because not every analysis is so enjoyable and because we don't always look forward to ending. Still, I'm quite sure that most of the time, termination is the wiser way to go. And the way we want to go.

I nevertheless want to open the possibility that in some instances the analytic story can have a sequel not only without ill effect, but in ways that enrich the patient's life. And every so often, in ways that also enrich the analyst's. We need to explore, rather than foreclose, this possibility by querying both our wish to continue our connection post-termination *and* our wish to end. To move post-treatment friendships out of the analytic closet and consider the possibility that they can reflect an achievement rather than a failure. To address the underside of the termination ideal, along with the complex problems that surface when we override it. In so doing, we move away from a problematic binary. We also honor two human needs—for nonneurotic, rich connection, as well as for separation.

# Part 3

# Beyond the Consulting Room

## Mourning, Actuality, and Illusions

# Introduction

Irwin Kula

Reading the last chapters of *Psychoanalysis and the Unspoken* is like watching a great veteran baseball pitcher use every piece of knowledge about the game acquired over a career to pitch a masterpiece. In chapters dealing with aging, mourning, loss, Covid, polarizing conflict, and self-doubt, Joyce Slochower doesn't simply leave the consulting room; she is *all in*. Drawing on her decades of knowledge as a theoretician and practitioner of psychoanalysis, Joyce shares her life experiences, specifically those that destabilize and overflow even her/our most adept ways of sense-making. The voices of the psyche are alive in each essay.

As I read these chapters, two images came to mind that I haven't thought about in decades. The first was the picture the late sociologist Peter Berger paints in the beginning of his great work, *The Sacred Canopy*. A child wakes up in the middle of the night terrorized by a nightmare, runs into her mother's room and, trembling, climbs into her bed. The mother, wakened, immediately holds her child close and says, "it's okay, it's okay, everything is going to be alright." And then Berger asks: "Is the mother lying?"

Of course, this is a secular koan. For even if everything goes incredibly well for this child, everything will not be alright. At the very best she will, one day, cry over the grave of the very person who told her, it's okay, everything will be alright. Joyce Slochower answers Peter Berger's question— is the mother lying—with a profound yes and an equally profound no.

The second is the last scene of the movie *The Truman Show* (a must watch for anyone reading this book!) when—spoiler alert—Jim Carrey (Truman) sails, in the most turbulent storm, toward the horizon and discovers that the ordered and beautiful world in which he has lived for decades is actually made up and constructed in its every interaction and detail by a maniacally controlling, creative, and compassionate movie director. His whole world has been an illusion, though he has lived his delightful life to

DOI: 10.4324/9781032691534-14

its fullest. We, the voyeurs of *The Truman Show* celebrate Truman's escape from illusion, but the movie ends without our knowing how Truman deals with his new "reality." In these last chapters, Joyce Slochower invites and models for us how to step out of the worlds made up by us and for us into an ever more real reality.

I am not a psychoanalyst. But Joyce and I have known each other for some thirty years. We help each other seek the truth about ourselves, others, and life and in the inevitable *collisions* that arise in relationships. I am the idealist grounded by Joyce's realism and Joyce the realist amused by my idealism. As Joyce comes out of the consulting room in these chapters, I—a seventh generation rabbi—long ago came out of the sanctuary to understand that the mystery of the depth of our psyche is as humbling, terrifying, compelling, inescapable, and unknowable as the gods of the heavens.

What is the through line of these chapters on aging, mourning, loss, Covid, polarizing conflict, and self-doubt? Surely, it is acknowledgment of our vulnerabilities and mortality, of the power, necessity, and limits of our illusions, of the inadequacy of all our theories and methods, of the ways we hold back, hold to, hold up and hold on for dear life, of the too muchness of reality—what William James calls the "flux" that inevitably blows up our rules, circuits, and conventions and melts (or rigidifies) the dualities with which we carve up reality to suit our human purposes. Joyce explores these themes with fierce grace. As I reread them, I experienced a celebration of finitude, a subtle revelation that we are finite beings yearning for the infinite, a trace of faith that stretches back to our ancestors (those we actively remember and those remembered in our DNA) and extends to the generations that we human beings can indeed get better at living.

In his song *Anthem*, Leonard Cohen reminds us that cracks in the bells are what allow the light in. Joyce cracks open the parts of life that are too hot to handle by whatever skillful means, wise theories, explicit or implicit metaphysics we possess . . . and light gets in.

In the chapter on aging, Joyce confronts how getting old, feeling our body weaken and our sexual allurement diminish, losing our memory, not having the same competencies nor the same energy to do life as we have lived it, informs, infiltrates, shapes, disrupts, traumatizes and, if not simply reframed and theorized, enriches life. In the chapter on mourning, Joyce lifts up the inadequacy of her own field of psychoanalysis and our contemporary culture in facing our need to mourn and evoke our losses across our lifetime. There is no "getting over," no final moving on, no letting go, no neat end point to remembering a loved one, no matter how together we are. Our deepest attachments and feelings are sustained across time. They transcend the borders of life and death and always have more to reveal. And so, Joyce turns her gaze on the personal, communal, and religious rituals that create space for interior processes to develop in their own way and time. She illustrates how they have helped to build the scaffolding that supports new relational and psychic capacities. In surrendering to absence, new forms of presence emerge.

In exploring the trauma around Covid, Joyce asks with unnerving honesty, what happens when we who are supposed to serve, tend, and heal others find our sense of safety, security, and order so disrupted and threatened that the illusions that buffer our existential anxieties are shattered? What do we do when our own subjectivity overwhelms our capacities and exceeds the power of the work we do? These are the actual experiences that interrupt and are qualitatively different from the regular flow of living and cannot be analyzed away! Here, Joyce's courage to wrestle with the too muchness of life shines through as she stays in a lived relationship with the rawness of reality and the unyieldingly disruptive and painful experience of a once in a lifetime plague.

There is such implicit trust and confidence here that speaking from where we are touched, from our own vulnerability and "unknowing," we not only birth new states of our own self but deepen our connection to those we serve. This is a cultural moment in which our body politic not only denies feelings of fear and shame that protect itself with a toxic certainty that has metastasized into demonizing and hurting others. Joyce's awareness that aliveness is dangerous, that as the Kabbalists teach, our vessels are always shattering, that in rejecting pain we inevitably amplify it person to person, family to family, culture to culture, that the central core of being alive has to do with the terror of annihilation, that only by making room for the deeper—and darker—processes of our psyches can we live together yet alone flourish—is no less than revelatory. To paraphrase the psalmist, "The beginning of wisdom is in the awe-fullness of UNKNOWING."

In the final chapters, Joyce navigates the polarization within the psychoanalytic community—and by implication our larger society—and takes on the self-doubt that comes with putting our ideas, our creativity, ourselves—on the line. Here, Joyce explores the challenge and need for a robust intellectual and psychological pluralism.

In the book of Genesis, we order the chaos and the overwhelmingness of reality, both the immenseness of the cosmos and the vastness of our inner space, by parsing and dividing things into binaries and polarities. Night and day, good and bad, us and them, sacred and profane, pure and impure, certainty and doubt, presence and absence, self and other, sameness and difference, obedience and transgression, being and doing. As inevitable as this way of mapping our reality is, it is always also a filtering, curating, reducing, dosing, simplifying of reality—a way to create predictability in the face of our fluidity, plurality, and contingency. As Joyce shows, we necessarily protect ourselves with theories and opinions that ensnare us on one side or another of these dualities; only if we re-integrate these binaries can we live more fully.

Can we develop the capacity to be open to and metabolize more of reality? Can we hold our truths, however self-defining, more lightly? Can we expand our ability to welcome, taste, process any kind of experience? Joyce makes room for complexity, multiplicity, and paradox, for the never-ending impact we have on each other and ourselves, for our yearning to be known and our fear of exposure, for the anxiety that comes with never arriving at final solutions to the challenge of knowing ourselves and being more deeply human.

These last chapters see life less as a journey from here to there than as a dance. A dance of chaos, order, and chaos, of forming, deforming, and reforming, of being lost and found and lost, of integrating, dis-integrating, and re-integrating, of figuring, dis-figuring, and re-figuring, of connecting, dis-connecting, and re-connecting, of being born, dying, and being reborn. Sometimes the dance is a waltz, sometimes a hora, sometimes a conga line and sometimes a whirling dervish of a dance. Joyce knows the steps.

I am writing this on the first day of the Hebrew month of Elul, one month before Rosh Hashana, the Jewish New Year. Beginning this morning and for the rest of this month, in synagogues around the world, the shofar—a ram's horn—will be blown in anticipation of Rosh Hashanah. The message of the blasts of the shofar: Wake Up, Grow Up, Show Up. These last chapters are like the blast of a shofar with accompanying wisdom.

Reading these chapters gives me a new understanding of the ninth of the Ten Commandments: Do Not Bear False Witness. Joyce comes out of the consulting room to beckon us to get better at *bearing witness* to our own and to each other's experiences. To become more truthful witnesses of our own subjectivity. To become better at seeing, listening, feeling with each other as the more we allow each other to unfold the less we will unravel. To never stop asking ourselves the very first two questions in the Torah:

Where are you?
Where is your brother?

I conclude with one last piece of Jewish wisdom. Why does the Torah end with Moses dying atop a mountain looking into, but not getting into, the Promised Land? Perhaps to teach us that there is no reaching the Promised Land. It remains forever promised, perpetually on the horizon, always being redefined even as approached. And the only real question is with whom we want to wander. These chapters reaffirm for me and will, no doubt, for you, how blessed we are to be wandering with Joyce Slochower.

# Chapter 9

# Getting better all the time?

Sam is divorced, in his late 40s. He speaks of his feelings about me, feelings that range from warm affection to anger. He also talks about sexual desire and erotic fantasies.

Sam's fantasies are mostly organized around an attractive female colleague. I listen for transference allusions, however indirect. For desire aimed my way. But I've yet to hear any. Sam's erotic fantasies—veiled or not—are not about me. Damn.

Feminism notwithstanding, it's painful to feel physically invisible. Of course, when I was younger and there was heat in the consulting room, this wasn't always easy either. I felt all kinds of things when my patients expressed sexual wishes toward me—desire, self-consciousness, anxiety. I tried to remain aware of the inadvertent seductive element embedded in transference exploration. There were days when I was careful to avoid low-cut tops and short skirts.

No more. These days I feel as sexually invisible to Sam as I am to the construction workers who would have whistled at my 20-year-old self. Then, I hated being objectified. But I hate being unseen just as much. It's a big narcissistic injury.

My young patients see me not as an object of sexual desire but instead as a sort of cool version of their mother—even their grandmother. But they are wont to say things like "Do you know about streaming music?" "Do you know what Instagram is?" I tend to feel mildly insulted by these questions. And I deal with them badly, I think; I joke, reassure them that I've indeed encountered the internet. Of course, sometimes I'm confronted with something I really don't know, something that dates me. And I feel slightly rattled.

On one hand, I am—and love being—a grandma. I didn't even mind (much) when my 5-year-old grandson asked me why the skin on my neck

DOI: 10.4324/9781032691534-15

was "crinkly." I didn't mind much because I adore him, not because I like my old neck. On the other hand, I live in a—partially fantasied—younger version of myself and my body. Not only don't I feel old, but I'm also surprised and offended when given a seat on the subway. I don't identify at all with Simon and Garfunkel's "Old Friends" who "sat on a park bench like bookends." After all, in the past two years I've hiked the Atlas Mountains, the Dolomites, and the French Alps. In summer, I regularly bike 30-plus miles. And I can leg press 230 pounds. Yes, I'm showing off. I collect comments about how fit I am with something close to glee. Those comments seem to negate the fact that, fit or not, I'm getting old. Is all this an adaptive version of the manic defense? A problematic one?

Probably both. Still, I think denial is underrated.

As I write this, I'm also acutely aware that 73 is not 83—or 93. That I'm far from done aging. That to my oldest colleagues, I'm still on the young side. So, I write as a younger old person who's now confronting getting really old for the first time.

I began writing about aging four years ago while in the Berkshires with good friends. Anticipating a challenging hike up a mountain while they took the sedate lake route, I felt like Tarzan. But then, a freak accident (and I underscore—defensively—an accident that wasn't my fault) shattered that illusion: A sticky boot sole stuck to the floor, and I fell hard on my kneecap. After a brief period of manic denial (I was sure it wasn't broken), I picked up my grandson at preschool and took him to his music class. I reassured a friend that we would, indeed, be flying out the following day for a vacation as planned. And hobbled back to my office to see a study group.

Midway through my study group, reality broke through. I was in acute pain and could no longer deny it. My group, with utter graciousness, helped me downstairs and into a cab that took me to urgent care. Yes, the patella had fractured. I had to cancel not only my trip but my patients and groups as well. In a straight leg brace for weeks, in considerable pain, unable to turn over in bed or walk easily, no less run or bike, the manic defense collapsed, and I got depressed. Flooded by a kind of PTSD triggered both by the unexpected fall and the helplessness I confronted, I struggled to work with my patients' responses.

To a person, my patients and supervisees were kind and solicitous. But beneath all this, there was more, of course. Only as I recovered did I learn how varied and complex were some patients' reactions to my injury. Concern, distress, annoyance, and, for one person, the reevocation of a trauma.

I soon refound my analytic self and, as I did, I also turned back to denial—walking more than I should, determined not to let my muscles atrophy. I paid for that, prolonging the recovery period. Still, two months later I was hiking in New Zealand, vulnerable no longer. For now.

## Analytic process outside time

There's something so utterly timeless about analytic process that it can be engaged to perpetuate an illusion of timeless intactness. We enter this work convinced we'll be there to see it through. Our investment in our therapeutic capacity makes it extraordinarily difficult to contemplate the loss of that capacity. I think this is true even though we identify the analyst's emotional vulnerability as core to therapeutic efficacy.

We psychoanalysts have mostly been silent on the subject of aging as it breaks into the illusion of timelessness. We've sidestepped the reality that helplessness and need will eventually infiltrate our lives and may well interfere with our capacity to do this work, that we'll eventually need help of one kind or another. Our sense of therapeutic agency and competence buffers what we know; many of us ignore/deny/disavow the loss of capacity—whether physical or cognitive—that's likely to surface down the road.

It's as if adults aren't vulnerable, only babies. Winnicott (1975) for example, spoke about the baby's need for a sustained sense of "going on being." Continuity of self exists only when massive impingements don't repeatedly disrupt. Impingements bring with them a threat of annihilation, but only for babies, or in instances of acute adult trauma (e.g., Boulanger, 2007). Neither Winnicott nor Melanie Klein (1948) considered our adult vulnerability to the *real* ending of our going on being.

Few of our psychoanalytic ancestors took up the question of our own ending. Frommer (2005, 2014, 2016) describes the history of early analysts' (e.g., Freud, 1923, 1926) failure to contend with our own mortality. Akhtar (2011) made a plea for us analysts to directly address the fear of dying. Arguing that death anxiety is not a dynamic derivative, he notes that,

> . . . as psychoanalysts, we have paid inoptimal attention to the psychological significance of the fact that all human beings die and that knowing this fact has enormous psychological ramifications. By ignoring,

bypassing, or downplaying this fact (and its undeniable, even if unconscious, dynamic impact), we have imbued life, living, physical health, analysis, and analyzing with a wishful hypomania.

(p. 121)

That "wishful hypomania" evades the inevitable and its dynamic consequences. It's as if, once we've matured and developed a solid sense of ourselves, we expect we'll deal easily with the deterioration and ultimately the loss of that very self. We idealize maturity, envision the equanimity with which we should face our own end. We assume that, if we're psychologically healthy, we'll manage our aging without rigidifying, becoming self-centered, much less despairing. That we'll grow old and move toward Erikson's (1950) generativity and ego integrity. That nurturing the next generation will be enough.

Toward the end of his life, Erikson (1984, 1998), in collaboration with his wife, Joan, added a ninth stage to his developmental model. This last stage addressed the challenges of old age. It, like the eighth stage, is organized around the tension between integrity, wisdom, and despair. But despair looms larger toward the end of life as we confront physical and cognitive deterioration and revisit all previous developmental stages.

> Epigenetically speaking, then, we can say that all the later age-specific developments are grounded or rooted in (and in fact dependent on) the strengths developed in infancy, childhood, and adolescence. And if the sense of autonomy "naturally" suffers grievously in old age, as the leeway of independence is constricted, there can also mature an active acceptance of appropriate limitations and a "wise" choice of involvements in vital engagements of a kind not possible earlier in life—and possibly (this we must find out) of potential value to a society of the future.
>
> (Erikson, 1984, p. 161)

Here, the Eriksons name what was sidestepped in the earlier—eight stages—model: The horror that aging and the prospect of death evoke. They provide us with an ideal worth aiming for—a capacity to face our own ending with wisdom and integrity. They also imply that we can use our wisdom to accept the painful losses old age brings with it.

Can we? *Is* it possible to encompass the actuality of our growing irrelevance, the loss of ourselves? The terror and deep grief connected with absence and absent connections to loved ones? I think not. No matter how realistically we accept our own progressive incapacity and, ultimately, our death.

A friend told me about such a moment of terror: He's 72, in good health, aware only of the minor cognitive slips many of us complain about. Then, at the end of a long and fatiguing workday, he opened his office door to invite his last patient in, only to realize that he had absolutely no access to her name. This wasn't a new patient either. Such a thing had never before happened, and he called me later in a panic. Is this the beginning of Alzheimer's? Of dementia? Merely a sign of fatigue? I wanted desperately to reassure him (and implicitly of course, to reassure myself). But I didn't know.

## Aging and dying

If we're lucky, aging will precede death by decades, decades that help us hold onto denial. If something breaks into our denial, it's usually illness. There's been a lot of excellent writing on illness in the therapist (e.g., Dewald, 1982; Friedman, 1991; Kahn, 2003; Morrison, 1997; B. Pizer, 2009). They and others movingly describe the impact of the analyst's physical vulnerability on therapeutic process. But physical illness represents a break in our ordinary "going on being." Aging doesn't. It's expected, it's part of life. But it's a part we work energetically to ignore.

In earlier psychoanalytic times, many analysts felt obliged to maintain therapeutic neutrality even when it required an active negation of reality. Decades ago, my friend's analyst continued working as lung cancer decimated her. Even though the analyst moved a hospital bed into the consulting room, she never acknowledged her illness to her patients; my friend knew she wasn't to say anything about what she saw. And so, her analyst's death arrived, unacknowledged and unprocessed.

I don't think this sort of thing happens often today. Our patients are freer to name what they see and we're more committed to addressing what's going on between us. But I'm not sure our capacity to confront the acute has much improved our engagement with ordinary aging. With its quieter iterations.

Here's a paradox: I've never felt better about my work. I trust my analytic intuition; I work deeply, and with far more ease than in earlier years. I have a sense of clinical wisdom that I certainly lacked as a young analyst. When I don't know what's going on, I can stay in the process without the kind of anxiety that plagues my younger supervisees. Yet it's also clear that aging has had other, less appealing effects. I can, for example, forget what I came into the room looking for, forget whether I've told someone something already or not. I can fail to record payments, or record one incorrectly. While I've always been a bit forgetful in these ways, I suspect I forget more often now; even if that's not the case, I get more anxious about it when I do. I try to preemptively manage my anxiety by owning my mistakes, sometime joking about the effects of aging on memory. My supervisees and patients smile, nod, and say little.

They too are invested in preserving my intactness.

It has always been tough for us analysts to hold our vitality in tension with our vulnerability, but perhaps never more than when we're confronting something irreversible. Will we have the guts to acknowledge that we're deteriorating? Will we find the courage to affirm our patient's concerns, or will we offer reassurance in the form of dynamic interpretations? "I'm fine, what's embedded in your anxiety?" "Do you worry that I'll leave you prematurely like your mother/father did?" "Is there a part of you that's waiting for me to go?"

## Not dealing with reality

In an essay on views of retirement among psychodynamically oriented psychiatrists, Ingram and Stine (2016) describe how reluctantly many respond to the prospect. Being asked "Are you still working?" feels insulting, ageist, a negation of our capacity. I feel this acutely; I barely restrain myself from snapping back when people assume I'm retired.

Most of us cannot fathom that we might want to retire, to do something different with our lives, and we avoid thinking seriously about retirement's meaning to us. We're so deeply identified with our work that losing it feels like the loss of self. Indeed, many of us declare that we'll work till we die. We sidestep the possibility that we might be forced to stop because we're ill or incapacitated. When infirmity of one kind or another does preclude our working, we confront the loss of our professional selves along with the loss of our patients. And since being an analyst means inhabiting a space where the personal and the professional interpenetrate, retirement represents a double loss.

A minority of us do choose to retire. We try to prepare our patients for termination and address its impact on them and on us. Still, this kind of leave-taking has profound relational implications. Retirement isn't something we arrive at in dialogue with our patient—we alone decide. Understandably enough, we're sometimes experienced as selfish and/or abandoning, especially, perhaps, when our retirement is a choice that's not forced upon us by illness. We're alive, we may even be quite well, but for our patient, there's no going back.

Our patients aren't replaceable either; closing a practice means losing multiple intimate connections. And even if there's relief at being free of the burden of a rigidly scheduled life and/or of ongoing responsibility for the other, loss, grief, and guilt may coexist (and be exacerbated by) that relief.

What makes it so hard for us to let go of this work? Is being an analyst especially compelling because it offers us something we rarely find outside the field—a kind of intimacy that's at once rich, satisfying, and yet protected by its asymmetry in a way that nonanalytic relationships are not (Frommer, personal communication, 2000)?

Whatever the particulars of our reason for not retiring, the shadow of mortality hangs over that choice. While I think this is true at every transitional life stage, it packs a particular punch when aging drives it (Chessick, 2013; Frommer, 2014; Hoffman, 1998, 2000). Frommer (2005, 2016) movingly describes the dynamics underlying our terror of mortality. McWilliams (2017) acknowledges our difficulty contending with mortality and also underscores the potential upside to aging. Nass (2015) challenges us to retire preemptively. But few of us take him up on that challenge (Ingram & Stine, 2016).

Our avoidance probably reflects both denial and the profound investment and satisfaction we derive from our work. But not thinking about retirement has a downside. It obscures, often forecloses, our need to think and plan. We don't seriously consider what else we might want or be able to do. Yes, many of us take more time off, but it's time *off*; it's not a different life.

Denial of aging can also affect us on a practical level. It's not uncommon for analysts to enter older age without the savings that would allow us to retire. Many of us don't have adequate pension plans; we continue to work because we need the income. I suspect there's some omnipotent denial lurking here; that denial, in tandem with actuality, can keep us working beyond the point when illness or cognitive deterioration infiltrate our clinical capacity. Will we have the wherewithal to acknowledge and explore our patients' response to this? Will we have the guts to retire because we must? Or will we soldier on, excluding what we can't bear to acknowledge?

My father was a psychoanalyst. In his mid-80s, he suffered several TIAs and some degree of cognitive impairment. I don't know how or when his patients ended treatment with him, or he with them. But I know that one did not, because shortly after my dad's death, a man phoned and asked to meet with me, having been sent my way by a caregiver. The former patient and I spoke at some length. When I asked him whether he had realized that my father's functioning was compromised, he said that he had, and, probably in response to my surprised look, added that being with him was "nevertheless a real comfort." He also indicated that my father hadn't addressed his failing health with him.

I wonder whether my father contemplated sending this man elsewhere. Did he consciously choose to continue the treatment out of awareness of this vulnerable patient's need for a relationship? Out of his own need—for the contact, the feeling of usefulness? I imagine that both derived comfort from this old connection, from being together. On one level, this was a mutual collusion, a denial of reality *and* an ethical breach. But on a human level, perhaps not only a bad thing.

How *do* we know when to retire? Is there an age when we should disqualify ourselves altogether even if we're well? When, for example, does minor forgetfulness bleed beyond tolerable borders? And what do we do about our patients' need not to see how old we are? Should we allow them to maintain an illusion of our invulnerability or alert them to our deterioration? To a chronic illness? Simply to the fact that we're getting old?

On one level, this is all way too concrete. After all, age is hardly perfectly correlated with death or with deterioration. Some of us age really well. I have a 101-year-old analyst friend (still in practice) who skied expert slopes until two years ago. She gives me hope. On the other side, young analysts get ill and die too. And freak accidents threaten us all. I think, with horror, of Jeremy Safran's tragic ending. Of Lew Aron's death at 66.

## Our theory and our aging selves

It's a platitude—and a sometimes truth—that with time and aging come wisdom and skill. Despite Winnicott's (1960b) warning that sometimes the new analyst, like the new mother, does a better job because she allows the patient to communicate what's needed before acting on her accrued knowledge, it's also true that experience counts a lot. Our clinical wisdom (Baum-Baicker, 2018; Baum-Baicker & Sisti, 2012) helps us become better analysts to our patients.

That aging—and time—affect clinical skill is self-evident. Less so is how, and if, it affects how we practice and how we think about what we do. Do we shift our theory or alter our adherence to it as we grow older? Do we become less theoretically rigid, or more so? Not wanting to lean too heavily on what's autobiographical, I spoke to 21 of my older colleagues and asked them how they see their clinical theory and use of it to have changed over time.

There was broad consensus that we're better analysts now than we were. We've been around the block; we're far more skilled—we're wiser, have better timing, more emotional resilience than we did in earlier years. We're more comfortable with our intuitive knowing because it's backed by decades of experience. We don't need to *find* theory before we move clinically because theory is in our bones. All this usually, but not always, makes us better analysts.

Aging can also bring with it a different kind of maturity linked to an intensified awareness of time and endings. We're more cognizant of life's limits, the actuality of lost opportunities, the inevitability of death, in a way that we weren't in our 40s.

All this is good—and not. On one hand, it helps us help people with their own existential anxieties, with the threat (or reality) of illness, aging, and dying—*if* we can deal with our fears. But it's also likely that our own existential anxieties will be activated along with our patients'. For those whose personal ghosts have been under-mourned and under-processed (Kalb, 2015), aging intensifies their presence. Awareness of lost opportunities, envy of younger patients and colleagues, regret in its many forms, foreclose a sense of generativity. We become preoccupied with our past and frightened of our future.

These preoccupations can affect our clinical work in worrisome ways. Some of us burn out, become bitter or deeply regretful about our own failures and losses, even go through the motions of being an analyst. We stop attending to clinical cues, to our patients' response to us. We avoid thinking about how our aging, our planned or unplanned retirement, affects them. Others create a barrier against regret by using patients in an attempt to enliven ourselves and preserve a sense of worth. We implicitly ask our patients to affirm our vitality as a wedge against anticipated loss; in the process, we exploit them emotionally.

Even for those who have mostly turned our ghosts into ancestors (Loewald, 1972), reality bites. It forces us to face the fact that we do *not* have all the time in the world, that analysis is *not* a sanctuary from life (Hoffman, 1998). Without the sanctuary element, we are really up against it—up against what we half thought would never happen to us. And I think this is true even for those of us who evade despair and remain self-reflective. A new kind of porousness disrupts the illusion that previously buffered existential anxieties; it's an illusion our patients help support because transference factors tend to shape their experience of us as robust and (at worst) middle-aged. And if we're seen as elderly, it's easy enough to chalk that up to our patient's projection rather than to reality.

Beyond the personal, aging often informs what we do in the clinical moment. While some of us keep getting better at it—more intuitive, wiser, more able to use ourselves—others rigidly live by old "shoulds" as a way of surviving analytically. We stick to the rules as a way of holding on for dear life.

More often, we let go of rules and get too loose. Therapeutic self-confidence forecloses self-reflectivity. We don't question what we're doing or why; we don't seek out supervision or peer consultation or pause much before we chat or self-disclose; we talk too much about ourselves. And we're less likely to pay close attention to the impact of those self-disclosures on our patient. I'm talking about a looseness that's not merely embedded in our theory or in a commitment to intersubjective engagement. It's a looseness that emerges out of a kind of disengagement from an earlier sense of therapeutic discipline. Perhaps also some self-indulgence. Both may reflect our intensified longing for contact, a longing informed by our awareness of the ticking clock.

The loss of a sense of timelessness also alters our perspective on analytic process. On one level, aging activates a quality of urgency. Some of us find it increasingly difficult to dwell comfortably in protected analytic space, to tolerate the slowness of the work. We want to help people change *now*, before it's too late, before we're/they're gone. We worry about our patients' denial—about the regret they'll feel when time and death end things. This worry can lend a palpable urgency to our clinical work. We're moved to engage more deeply and to push harder.

But aging pulls others toward more equanimity about the slowness of analytic process. A longer view helps us accept the limits of people's capacity to change and leaves us more content with subtle movement. We become less ambitious about what we aim to achieve and less impatient when change seems glacial. Most of my colleagues noted that the two threads of urgency and equanimity, while omnipresent, affect them differently depending on the particulars of each treatment relationship.

However aging affects us in the consulting room, there was wide agreement that aging activates a sense of urgency in our personal lives. We begin to privilege our own desires; after all, it's now or never—the day is coming when we won't be able to undertake that arduous trip we've been dreaming about forever. Most of us feel less willing to take on patients whose needs bleed into evenings and weekends. We take more vacation than ever. Some of us move away from three- and four-times-a-week analyses; working at lower frequencies gives us more freedom, literal and emotional. But others feel energized by the affective aliveness of more intense work and seek it out.

Whether aging insulates us emotionally *or* activates our sense of vulnerability, it shifts our relationship to, and awareness of, our own needs as they collide with our patients'. The unconscious becomes less timeless (Loewald, 1972)—the desire and fear it contains break into our awareness. This can manifest in different ways, but often leaves more of "us" informing the clinical and personal choices we make.

Aging also shifts our self-experience in the clinical moment, though in variegated ways. One colleague sees herself to be in a kind of existential place, a bit removed from the emotional pressures that used to feel quite intense. She thinks she's less susceptible to the attacks leveled at her by her borderline patients and that this makes her a better, less reactive analyst. But another colleague feels more vulnerable than ever and is less able/willing to tolerate work that can destabilize things; he refers very disturbed people elsewhere. A third sees time as having matured him; he's less likely to go on the interpretive offensive. Awareness of his aging leaves him feeling that he and they are "like subjects" with whom he can identify.

Often, of course, our patients age along with us. A colleague notes that work with his oldest patients frequently focuses on shared existential anxieties—the reality of losing ground, of illness, loss, and death. He remarked in passing that the kind of wisdom his patients need from him is not to be found in our psychoanalytic canon (Frommer, personal communication, 2018). And I agree.

Along with maturity can come a shift in the identifications evoked in us. In earlier years, when a patient described her parents as remote, withholding, or hostile, my instinct was to empathize with that description rather than to challenge it overtly or privately. No longer; at least, not reflexively. Now my identification tends to go the other way, toward the patient's parents and sometimes the grandparents.

I have a somewhat irritable reaction to clinical presentations that provide one-word descriptions of a patient's parent as, for example, "narcissistic" or "cold." I'm reacting to the stereotype, to the oh-so-easy, one-off dismissal of parental subjectivity.

I'm also being differently defensive. It's so much easier for me to get the parental side, to feel the immaturity of the grown-up child, her insensitivity to her parent. Yes, like my own grown children, at times.

And so, when my 47-year-old patient bitterly complains that his 80-year-old mother made "the outrageous demand that I drive the family down to visit her rather than having her come to visit us," I feel both mildly alarmed and mildly judgmental. I want to address his conflicted negation of their attachment *and* of his mother's vulnerability. Not merely because his defensiveness forecloses much that he feels. I'm also acutely aware that time is running out for her—and for them. I want to help him repair his relationship to his mother before it's too late.

Losing the sanctuary element can move me away from a focus on dynamics and toward a focus on "reality." When my 75-year-old patient talks about his awareness that this next overseas trip may be his last, that he can't count on remaining intact, I don't have even a momentary wish to interpret his awareness as defensive or anxiety driven.

I say, simply, "I know."

## How does our theory age?

It's not only we who have aged. Psychoanalytic theory has as well; it's more complex, more flexible, less authoritarian. It explicitly addresses the intersubjective element. I think this is true whatever the particulars of our theoretical identification. In part, these theoretical shifts have contributed to the shift we ourselves make as we age.

With time, we metabolize aspects of our clinical position. As it becomes ours, we move away from a reflexive reliance on it and shape an implicit theory of therapeutic action that's more procedural than deliberate. And often more flexible.

Like most of my older colleagues, I've stopped consulting my analytic superego about what I can and can't say or do, about answering questions and the like. This often means I've loosened up, am less rule-bound. But I'm also more comfortable and less conflicted about drawing what feels like a necessary line. Yes, these shifts mirror the sociocultural, personal, and psychoanalytic sea change away from authoritarianism and toward asymmetrical mutuality (Aron, 1991). But they also reflect clinical experience and maturity—often, but not necessarily—correlated with aging.

My work bridging Winnicottian and relational theory took shape several decades ago—when I really was younger. In many ways, I stand behind this vision; it makes room for my patient's affective resilience—or vulnerability—over an insistently relational, confrontational, or interpretive stance. It creates space and allows interior process to develop in its own way and time. I can be myself *and* privilege my patient's needs.

But as I've aged, I've also shifted a bit away from this theoretical tilt. That shift has been both procedural and theoretical. Here's the procedural part: My classical and object relational analytic training left me a somewhat rule-bound, anxious young analyst, and it took several decades, more analysis, and lots of clinical experience before I got over much of that. Additionally, I've become less enamored of my own theory of holding (Chapter 5). I'm more aware of the ways that holding and intersubjectivity interpenetrate. And time has, to some extent, eroded my willingness to ongoingly bracket my subjectivity.

I've also become more cognizant of, and somewhat more cautious about, the potential underbelly to four-times-weekly analysis and regression to dependence as therapeutic linchpins. Certainly, holding and regression allow some patients to refind and rework early trauma in an analytic context that repairs. All this can be a good—indeed, a crucial—thing, therapeutically speaking. But regression has an underbelly. My regressed patient has something (sometimes a lot) to lose in the present. Her job, relationship, sense of intactness may be on the line. And so today, I think more than I did about helping my patient develop her own capacities—for "doing" and for affect regulation; that is, her resilience. Embedded here is my awareness that I won't be around forever.

Do most of us become more theoretically flexible over time? Do we move away from a belief in our therapeutic efficacy and toward a focus on helping patients develop more resilience? Or do some of us move the other way—toward a fuller embrace of our own reparative capacity as a wedge against a sense of diminishment? I suspect there's evidence for both threads, depending on a range of personal dynamic factors.

Here's what I do think is usually true: Over time—that is, as we age—we tend to shift our relationship to the theory on which we've relied. While some of us abandon or rewrite our theory, more often we both complicate it and loosen our attachment to it. It's easier for us to allow multiple theoretical narratives to coexist because we no longer feel the need to choose or pledge allegiance.

It's impossible to parse the role of time (aging), changes in the psychoanalytic sensibility of our cohort, and clinical experience in this shift. There's not much literature on how our clinical theory changes over time, and certainly the perspective of 21 clinicians is an inadequate sample. I offer these thoughts to get you to think about the question. If you're old. But also if you're not. Because, hopefully, one day you will be.

# Chapter 10

# Out of the analytic shadow

As I discuss in Chapter 9, aging confronts us with potential—and actual—loss. What helps us encompass those losses that cannot be analyzed away?

Something other than psychoanalysis. We need to leave the consulting room when we mourn actual loss (as opposed to symbolic or dynamically driven loss). Culturally and religiously derived bereavement rituals provide us with something that psychoanalysis cannot. But we don't often explore the dynamic function of these rituals because of the heavy ideology with which they're laden (Ashenburg, 2002). Here, I describe and theorize the therapeutic function embedded in these non-psychoanalytic practices using my personal experience with Jewish mourning and memorial ritual to illustrate.

## Loss, mourning, and *shiva* ritual

It wasn't until my own father died that I encountered mourning ritual first-hand. His sudden death left me shocked; yes, he was 90, but he had been well the night before he died. There was no warning, no opportunity to say goodbye, no last hug, just a phone call announcing his death. Unable to encompass his death, grief-stricken, I wanted only to be with family and my closest friends, not strangers or acquaintances.

I sat *shiva* reluctantly and was more than a little surprised to find the experience to be profoundly therapeutic.

## Death and mourning

All cultures recognize the mourner's need to honor the deceased and express grief at the loss (Mandelbaum, 1959), and every culture (and

DOI: 10.4324/9781032691534-16

religion) has developed commemorative rituals to mark and support the grieving process. While only religious Jewish communities scrupulously observe the laws of mourning, many secular Jews have incorporated aspects of *shiva* and *yizkor* ritual into mourning observance, though in a truncated way (e.g., by sitting *shiva* for three days rather than seven). That shouldn't be surprising. Contemporary culture approaches death gingerly; it can seem easier to simply get on with life and relegate traditional mourning observance to an earlier time and place. Yet both mourning and memorial ritual can have a powerful therapeutic impact on the mourner. I begin with *shiva*.

While mainly orthodox Jews observe these practices in all their detail, aspects of *shiva* observance can be found in nonorthodox Jewish tradition as well. Whatever the particulars, *shiva* has the potential to create a holding environment for the mourner. Here I outline central *shiva* tradition; see Lamm (1988) for a thorough summary.

In Jewish tradition, one sits *shiva* for only parents, siblings, children, and spouse—the most central and least replaceable in life. The first stage of mourning (*aninut*) begins at the moment of death when the mourner's loss is concretized by making a tear in the mourner's outer garment (*keriah*). This dramatic act both reenacts the mourner's torn state and symbolically separates the mourner from the world.

From death until burial, the body is physically accompanied by a silent observer, ideally a member of the mourner's community. Shortly before burial the body is bathed, dressed, and placed in a casket, sometimes by members of the mourner's own community. Burial itself has a stark impact; an unadorned wooden casket (or, in Israel, a shroud without a casket) is used. At the cemetery, the coffin or shroud is covered with earth by the mourner(s), the mourner's family, and the community.

*Shiva* itself begins when the mourner returns home from the cemetery. The mourner washes hands prior to entering the home (this symbolizes a cleansing following contact with death). Mirrors (associated with vanity) are covered. A symbolic meal of condolence is traditionally provided by the community, and includes foods associated with life, such as bread and hard-boiled eggs. A memorial (*yahrzeit*) candle is lit; it will burn for the seven-day *shiva* period.

S*hiva* traditions disrupt ordinary social behavior for both mourner and visitor. These disruptions, at once socially awkward *and* therapeutically central, establish powerful barriers against superficial social interchange and symbolically embody the mourner's state of grief and separation from the community. For example, in orthodox communities, many mourners don't wear leather shoes[1] (traditionally associated with comfort and vanity) or study Torah (such study is believed to bring joy). Some refrain from shaving, using cosmetics, cutting hair, or engaging in sexual relations. They neither bathe (unless they find this restriction very difficult) nor change clothing, particularly the rent garment. Mourners sit on a low stool or chair[2]; they aren't expected to rise, greet, or otherwise entertain the caller. These customs create a protected space that offers few distractions from the loss experience.

Visitors to the mourner operate under similarly unusual traditions. A *shiva* call is considered its own good deed and obligation (*mitzvah*). Callers generally come unannounced at any time during the day or evening; thus, for much of the day, the mourner is with others whose sole purpose is to provide comfort. The mourner may speak about the loss, share memories of the deceased, or avoid the subject of loss altogether.

The caller, who isn't expected to stay long, doesn't say goodbye. Some utter a traditional phrase, "May God comfort you among the mourners of Zion and Jerusalem." Others make statements like "May we meet on a happier occasion," acknowledging the mourner's grief but bridging present and future by suggesting that life will again bring joy. The mourner isn't expected to acknowledge the caller's statement but remains seated, i.e., remains the mourner.

On the morning of the seventh day, the mourner is traditionally escorted on a short walk, a symbolic reentry into the world outside the home. Although the mourner then "gets up" from *shiva* and resumes daily life in most respects, traditional observance continues during the subsequent 30 days (*shloshim*) and certain activities (such as attending parties, concerts,

---

1 These prohibitions originally involved not wearing shoes at all and sitting anywhere other than the floor. The ancient mourner was thus placed in close emotional and literal proximity to the deceased (Tractate Semachot, 6:1).
2 Contrary to popular belief, the chair need not be hard or uncomfortable. Instead, this low seat symbolizes the mourner's lowered emotional state.

etc.) designed to bring joy are curtailed. Many male mourners refrain from shaving throughout *shloshim*. An unshaven face represents a most powerful and visible expression of this bereaved state. In the instance of a parent's death (a loss lacking the possibility of even partial replacement), many male mourners (and increasingly, female mourners as well[3]) concretely acknowledge their loss by saying *kaddish* (mourner's prayer) in synagogue daily and limiting social activities and festivities for eleven months.

### Shiva's dynamic function

The laws of *shiva* are most complex; I've provided only a very broad outline here (see D. Kraemer, 2000). And because *shiva* occurs within a social and not an analytic context, its psychological meaning for the individual mourner is largely impenetrable. Certainly, my own response to my parents' *shiva* was subjective, colored both by my relationship to my father (and later, my mother) and my personal response to these traditions.

From the moment of my father's death, I felt at once profoundly alone *and* embedded in a holding community. When I went to the funeral home to arrange for my father's burial, I was moved to tears by the sight of a synagogue member with whom I was only slightly acquainted sitting with the body until the burial. At my mother's funeral, a decade later, a very close friend prepared the body. Thinking of her caring hands bathing my mom transformed a traumatic process into one of comfort.

At the cemetery, I found something both raw and compelling as we shoveled earth onto the plain pine casket. There was no possibility of denying death and its shock was intense. I then returned home to a meal prepared for me and my family. Having anticipated that I wouldn't want food, I was overwhelmed by the beautifully prepared meal (one of many to follow) that had been left for me—to eat or not as I chose. This provision carried with it no expectation of acknowledgment; it was both a symbolic and literal holding.

I remained at home for the week, both protected from and deprived of the external distractions that might be viewed as relieving the pain of

---

3  The custom of reciting the mourner's *kaddish* daily was (like all public prayer) traditionally viewed as a male obligation in the orthodox community but not in conservative or reform synagogues. Today, some orthodox women have also taken on this ritual.

loss; I neither worked, nor shopped, cooked for myself or my family, etc. Yet I was far from alone; a stream of *shiva* callers appeared who allowed me to talk about my father when I needed to and about other things when I did not. Visitors came and left unrequested, freeing me from the burden of having to ask for company that I didn't know I needed; at the same time, they made it possible for me to retreat in privacy when I needed to do so.

While some *shiva* callers were close friends or relatives, many were more casual acquaintances. To my great surprise, I was deeply touched by a stranger's visit—the mother of my son's friend—who entered and silently sat down. When I looked inquiringly at her, she identified herself, said no more, but sat quietly listening. Today, more than 30 years later, I feel grateful to her.

*Shiva* callers rarely interrupted me to share similar experiences ("when *my* father died . . ."); my state of acute mourning left me unable to make use of this kind of "like subject" linkage. Their traditional farewell greeting offered the comfort of community ("May God comfort you among the mourners . . ."). Even the awkward apologies of those unable to recite the somehow difficult phrase felt comforting; intention mattered more than form.

There were other ways of offering comfort as well—silent hugs, references to a future with other celebrations. Yes, we would all suffer painful losses, but we would also celebrate our kids' *bar* or *bat mitzvahs*, weddings, new babies. Hope was affirmed but not used to negate pain. I emerged from this intense week of remembering both exhausted and relieved. My recovery didn't end there, but was steady, supported by the love and care of family and friends.

*Shiva*, then, makes the denial of death impossible. Grief (whether felt or unfelt at any moment) is multiply embodied: My shoes, clothing, lowered chair, unadorned skin, etc., underscored my state of mourning and interfered with the possibility of "putting on a face" (false self) to the world. Yet very little was expected of me: I received callers' visits and farewells in silence. The custom requiring that the caller waits for me to speak first, strikingly akin to the opening of a therapy session, placed the emotional tone and content of the conversation in my hands and made it harder for any of us to escape into social convention.

### *Shiva's* holding function

*Shiva* thus creates an emotionally protective setting that's remarkably reminiscent of the therapeutic holding environment (Slochower, 1995, 2010; Winnicott, 1964). Like the parent or analyst whose protective presence permits the baby/patient a space in which to "go on being," during *shiva,* the mourner is the single subject in the room. It's the community of callers, rather than a single individual, that does the holding; it becomes a group of non-impinging witnesses who allow the mourner to use others without regard for their own needs (i.e., ruthlessly; Winnicott, 1965, 1971).

These rituals have the potential—not always reached—to create a transitional space characterized by paradox (Modell, 1990; S. A. Pizer, 1992; Winnicott, 1971). For a limited and circumscribed time and in a fixed setting, the *shiva* caller functions in a rather artificial way with a person acutely, but temporarily, in need. This space offers the mourner a non-regressive opportunity to experience and work through loss.

Even more than the analytic setting—which also takes place in a fixed place and at a set time—the boundary around *shiva* is quite rigid; the conclusion of the *shiva* week marks the absolute end of the caller's responsibility toward the mourner. Yet like the patient and analyst, mourner and caller don't ordinarily challenge the meaningfulness of *shiva.* Instead, there's an implicit agreement *not* to challenge its transience or the illusion of attunement characteristic of it but rather to tolerate its ambiguities.

### *Shiva's* intersubjective element

It's not always easy to pay a *shiva* call; this socially awkward tradition can be quite emotionally charged even when the loss isn't our own. Few of us have fully assimilated our feelings about death; paying a *shiva* call confronts us with our own unmetabolized feelings of anticipated or remembered deaths in our own life. Callers feel all kinds of things during a *shiva* call—empathy, anxiety, awkwardness, a sense of burden or discomfort about the mourner's need. Will the caller's response provide a holding function for the mourner, or will it become an emotional interference (impingement), derailing the mourner's inner process much as the analyst's expression of her subjectivity sometimes derails the patient (Chapter 4)?

While a grieving mourner easily evokes empathy and concern in the caller, it's more difficult to know what to say or how to "be" with a mourner whose grief is apparently absent. Some mourners' need to defend against grief appears as a flat focus on the self or on superficial matters. The caller may feel emotionally obliterated, useless, or awkward, even judgmental of the mourner's apparent lack of grief. Or relieved at the absence of emotional pressure. These feelings parallel the analyst's response to work with narcissistic patients (Modell, 1975, 1976).

When the mourner is conflicted about the loss or contends with guilt about past actions or inactions, hatred, or envy toward the dead person (cf. Klein, 1975), *shiva* ritual has a more complex effect: The caller's expressed concern may provoke guilt or anger in the mourner. Like the analyst working with an angry or self-blaming patient, the caller may want to withdraw out of hurt, annoyance, or anxiety.

When the mourner and/or the community can't tolerate the emotional strain of the holding process, *shiva* will fail. I vividly remember attending a *shiva* when those present (who were unfamiliar with mourning tradition) sat in strained silence interspersed with small talk and self-conscious political comments as they ate a meal provided by the mourners. Expressions of grief were foreclosed and *shiva* offered no relief at all.

At other times, it's not the community's emotional limitations that fail the mourner, but the traditions of *shiva* themselves. *Shiva* observance is limited to four categories of relationship (parent, spouse, siblings, and child). It excludes the deaths of loved ones who fall into different relationship categories (and infants under 30 days old). These losses leave the mourner without easy access to this holding space.

The holding function of the seven-day *shiva* period is also interrupted by *shabbat*. This one-day interruption may begin to draw the mourner back into life, much as small disruptions in holding can facilitate an integrative process in a patient. More problematic are times when a death coincides with a major holiday that (depending on precisely when the actual mourning begins) postpones or even cancels the *shiva* period. Here, the mourner's need to grieve is overridden by religious beliefs about the community's obligation to celebrate the holiday. If this failure in adaptation was preceded by a period of good-enough holding, it may be strengthening rather than traumatic. But when *shiva* is cut off in its early stages or canceled altogether, the mourner will likely be failed in a major way. I doubt that even a very observant mourner can fully suspend or bracket grief because of the religious obligation to celebrate a holiday. It's more likely that the mourner will feel traumatically unprotected. I've worked with several patients who had this reaction to a death that wasn't marked by *shiva* observance in contrast to their fuller mourning process where death was followed by *shiva*. (In Chapter 11, I discuss mourning during the Covid era.)

## What protects the caller?

Although *shiva* is designed to support the mourner, the caller's needs are implicitly embedded in *shiva* ritual in ways not unlike the protection provided the analyst by therapeutic parameters: *Shiva* calls are short, ordinarily paid only once by any individual; the holding function thus falls lightly on the individual caller. And although the caller allows the mourner to set the tone and content of the conversation, it's the caller, not the mourner, who decides when to visit and when to leave, expressing, perhaps, latent hatred in this way (Winnicott, 1949).

On the seventh day of *shiva*, the mourner "gets up," whether she's emotionally ready or not, thereby freeing the caller from further obligation. Further, because *shiva* observance is interrupted by *shabbat* and canceled by major holidays, the community's involvement in life supersedes the needs of the individual mourner. Like the analyst who ends sessions and takes vacations despite the patient's need for treatment, *shiva* tradition places the mourner's needs within a larger context of communal need. I suspect that these limits are what permit the community to tolerate the very great demand inherent in *shiva* observance.

In describing *shiva*'s potential therapeutic function, I've focused on the ideal. But it's not uncommon for *shiva* to fail the mourner because the mourner and/or the community cannot tolerate the discomfort generated by the ritual. And, of course, *shiva* requires community, something missing for too many. What's nevertheless compelling is the power of *shiva* ritual to meet an individual's temporarily intense need for a holding experience in its varied aspects, while still protecting the larger group.

## After *shiva*: Memorial ritual across a lifetime

Psychoanalysts long assumed that the grief following a death would gradually fade as the lost object is internalized. Mourning, it was thought, should be followed by working through and decathexis (Freud, 1914), not sustained, affect-laden remembering. Indeed, classical writers view prolonged grief as evidence of unresolved conflict and pathological mourning (Akhtar &

Smolar, 1998). But Loewald (1962, 1976) moved our thinking away from decathexis by underscoring the mourner's need to internalize rather than relinquish the object. From this perspective, the capacity to sustain an inner attachment to deceased loved ones is less pathological than integrative (Gaines, 1997; Klass, 1988; Lobban, 2007; Rubin, 1985; Shabad, 2001; Silverman, Nickman, & Worden, 1992).

Yet despite this shift and the privileged place psychoanalytic theories accord memory and grief, we rarely explore the dynamic function of commemorative ritual. Indeed, like religion (Freud, 1927), ongoing acts of mourning and memorial are traditionally viewed as a sign of psychopathology, as regressive rather than integrative. We tend to hear repetitive remembering as evidence of massive trauma, unresolved loss, conflict, or guilt, to be worked through rather than enacted and from which our patient will ultimately emerge. We aim for separation, hoping to help release our patients from the weight of loss, to free them (and ourselves) from the binding encumbrances of early, conflicted ties. We valorize, indeed idealize, "moving on" and "letting go." We believe in our capacity to leave the past behind.

The ideal of separation collides rather directly with those embodied in acts of memorialization. For commemorative rituals are aimed neither at decathexis nor at moving on, but instead at countering the absence created by death by reevoking loss and attendant, affect-laden memories. Commemorative ritual establishes a space of linkage, of "like subjects" (Benjamin, 1995a)—indeed, "like mourners"—and facilitates the construction of group memory.

The few psychoanalytic papers on memorialization explore its function for victims of massive trauma. These acts of commemoration often take place at the site of physical memorials, such as the Vietnam Veterans Memorial wall in Washington, D.C., Yad Vashem in Israel, and similar memorials worldwide (Homans & Jonte-Pace, 2005). Memorial sites have the potential to function as symbolic grave markers, "missing tombstones" (Ornstein, 2008), or shared linking object (Volkan, 1981)[4]. Although psychoanalysis has given such experiences short shrift, there are rich sociological and historical literatures on collective memory, particularly among

4 While memorial sites can usefully evoke loss, they can also block the process of remembering (Bassin, 1998, 2008; Volkan, 2007).

scholars of Jewish history (Halbwachs, 1992; Nora, 1984–1992, 1989; Yerushalmi, 1982; Zerubavel, 1995). What remains to be explored is the intrapsychic impact of commemorative rituals and their role in instances of "ordinary," rather than traumatic, loss.

We psychoanalysts have been somewhat suspicious of mourning and commemorative ritual, probably because they're usually embedded within cultural and religious practices that have strong—and alien—ideologies (Hagman, 1995a, 1995b). Yet we're hardly averse to ritual itself; on the contrary, analytic work uses more than a few rituals of its own. Quiet more than flamboyant, our psychoanalytic rituals (Hoffman, 1998) are lodged in the predictable, organized practices that shape therapeutic time, place, physical position, how we begin and end the session, and so on. We witness our patient's remembering, and together we co-create a wide memorial space within therapeutic walls.

But this kind of memorialization is a by-product of analytic process, for we don't structure sessions with commemoration as a goal; acts of "doing" have a very small place in psychoanalytic work; we abhor what's prescribed, including the deliberate evocation of specific affect states and memories, or explicit attempts to stimulate intragroup connectedness. Indeed, analytic ritual aims to minimize externally generated evocation and maximize access to interior experience. While as witnessing analysts we sometimes participate in our patient's remembering, therapeutic process tilts us toward the former function; it's our patient—not protocol—who shapes the session's content and the process of remembrance. If there's an element of commemorative action embedded within psychoanalytic process, then, it's more implicit than performative.

Essentialized, the very notion of commemorative ritual collides with the psychoanalytic relationship to time. For although we work within a treatment space buffered by an illusion of timelessness (Hoffman, 2000), we also assume—and rely on—the existence of a constructed ending. Indeed, termination is both the fate and goal of psychoanalytic process (Chapter 8). The considerable literature on termination (Bergmann, 1988, 1997; Pedder, 1988; Salberg, 2010) focuses largely on what facilitates (or impedes) the relinquishment and internalization of the analytic relationship. From this perspective, commemorative ritual reflects an underlying and problematic resistance to facing loss, a resistance to be analyzed rather than enacted.

Yet feelings of absence often remain with us across the lifespan. And I'm convinced we need periodic ways to honor personal losses. That need takes us beyond psychoanalysis; it can be found in multiple socially, culturally, and religiously constructed commemorative practices. Mexicans observe the Day of the Dead; Roman Catholics celebrate Mass; Muslims read a portion of the *Koran*; Jews observe *yahrzeit,* say *kaddish* and *yizkor.* Others engage in personal acts of remembrance; an annual visit to a cemetery; an afternoon spent with the photographs, books, letters, and songs of earlier times; yearly visits to the family home or town. These acts help shape the individual's memories of—and inner relationship to—the deceased by countering *and* reevoking the absence created by death.

## Loss and grief over time

My own understanding of memorial ritual coalesced around personal confrontations with loss. My parents were elderly when they died and I was middle-aged, so I'm among the fortunate. I escaped the extraordinary suffering of those who lose loved ones in childhood, horrific accidents, disease, war, or acts of terrorism. But we don't experience death comparatively. Both my parents' deaths were unexpected, and, in both instances, I was unprepared; their deaths disrupted, indeed, dismantled my own illusions—of timelessness, of my going on being their child forever. Both times I sat *shiva,* worked over the grief and regret with which I struggled, was comforted by my children and friends. Gradually, I emerged and got on with life. Their deaths, and the grief I felt, faded. But the insulation created by time was never thick. It was easily pierced—by the first *bar mitzvah* without my dad; by the first child's wedding without even one grandparent. In each instance, the acute awareness of a hole returned: I am now the oldest generation.

The porous nature of that insulation fueled my wish, more intermittent than chronic, to formally remember and honor my parents across time. I was in a good treatment during some of those years and had help working through these losses. However, I wanted and needed something more, and found it in memorial ritual.

Like *shiva, yizkor* is a religiously embedded memorial tradition. While it's unsurprising that Orthodox Jews observe *yizkor,* it's notable that 60 percent of nonorthodox American Jews make a point of attending only this portion of the synagogue service (Bethamie Horowitz, personal communication, 2009). *Yizkor* literally means "he will remember," but more colloquially is understood as remembering or remembrance. This act of memorial takes place during four major annual holidays, including *Yom Kippur*. Although anyone can recite *yizkor* in memory of those whose losses leave no family, it's ordinarily said for parents, siblings, spouse, or child. There's no end point to *yizkor* ritual; it's recited across the lifetime.

The *yizkor* service varies rather widely as a function of subculture and Jewish denomination; my own experience is primarily with the American Conservative Jewish tradition. That tradition has used a free hand in both following and embellishing the ancient liturgy by introducing innovations that enhance its emotional power.

*Yizkor* falls about halfway through the synagogue service. Because many people arrive just for this ritual, synagogues become unusually packed at this point. Although most of the service unfolds fluidly, *yizkor* is always announced; this gives people who haven't lost a close relative an opportunity to leave the room, to reaffirm the "real" relationship with loved ones. Yet leaving the room for *yizkor* is its own enactment, implicitly both denying (Becker, 1973) *and* acknowledging the idea of death. Loss, then, is in the air for all.

At *yizkor*, the low buzz accompanying much of the service stops (synagogue congregations are almost never entirely quiet). The mood grows solemn. A psalm is chanted and separate memorial prayers for individual loved ones are read silently; the name of each lost loved one is inserted into a separate version of the prayer. A memorial prayer is often followed by *kaddish*, and a concluding psalm is sometimes sung communally.

Until need and loss brought me into memorial space, the affective power of *yizkor* remained somewhat elusive, the words of the prayers stilted and a bit formulaic.

That changed after my father's death and intensified after my mother's.

Moments before *yizkor* was announced, I had been quietly chatting with a friend. Now, I settled into myself. Suddenly alone in the crowded room, I became immersed in painful memories of my mother's recent death. This was the hole of traumatic loss and there was no relief in memorializing her. I didn't so much read the requisite words; I used them as a window into a different emotional space and wept. But this wasn't the prolonged grief of mourning, only a very brief touching of it. For moments later, pulled along by the sound of turning pages and the awareness that I also wanted to say *yizkor* for my father, I moved away from the acuteness of recent loss and entered a quieter, sadder place, colored by nostalgia and a flood of memories. He's gone almost two decades, missed the *bar* and *bat mitzvahs* he longed to attend, my children's weddings, so many seders. He would have been delighted to see his grandchildren grow into adulthood. My father suddenly became alive, filled empty memory spaces as I contemplated what might have been. All of this in less than 10 minutes!

This, my first experience saying *yizkor* for both parents, didn't become a blueprint for the ritual; it continues to shift across time. At the risk of telescoping and flattening what has been a complex journey, I identify two dominant paths; one involves reexperiencing and reworking core affect states associated with loss and the second, the rediscovery and reshaping of associated memories.

Some years ago on *Yom Kippur*, I found myself musing about my son's wedding, which had recently taken place at the country home my father built. Caught up short by a visual memory of the ceremony, I suddenly realized that it took place on the very patch of lawn where, decades earlier, then a small child, I had watched my father clear the trees. Though I turned to the memorial prayer I always read for my maternal grandmother, my thoughts lingered over that space, and I recalled a photo of her holding me in a lawn chair as an infant. Reimagining that moment, I contacted a body memory of her chair, its soft canvas feel, an echo of my grandmother's soft arms around me.

I'm describing the recapturing of an affective experience that had been inaccessible till then. But more importantly, a new memory sequence coalesced and shaped a different narrative, a personal story of my relationship to place and person. It allowed me to link my grandmother to my father, to me, and to my children, who barely knew her. And with that linkage came a sense of restoration, as if I had invited my grandmother into her grandchild's wedding, back into my life.

Perhaps because I'm not ordinarily immersed in the past, *yizkor* provides an opportunity to go where I rarely do, to recontact old self-states, old relationships, and to bridge the very distant past by imbuing it with affect. I'm describing the use of narrative to restore and rework emotional memory within a protected holding space. I experienced absence and then filled it with presence, with a reconstructed image of old object ties.

The trajectory of this new relational memory space is softer and more nostalgic, but it's no less imbued with content. Now I mostly remember the parents of my childhood and less their aging and deaths. My father's gentle adoration, his Yiddish and German lullabies, although I haven't forgotten his sometimes-irascible temper. Memories of my mother have also shifted. I increasingly remember her earnestness and loving reliability. In writing this chapter, I recovered the memory of her singing a lullaby to me at bedtime, her easy and generous response to a shy request I made at age 7 or so for a white blouse with a Peter Pan collar that the "popular girls" wore. I still weep when I remember how she longed to dance at my son's wedding. But I now also can contact her delight as she danced with my 2-year-old daughter summers ago.

I suspect that acts of memorialization evoke a core psychoanalytic anxiety—that we never do lose our need for the other or our need to rework old connections—that we cannot fully separate, cannot fully terminate.

## From the interior toward the intersubjective

Mourning rituals like *shiva* establish a protected holding space within which to mourn. But as we return to our lives and away from traumatic loss, we reenter the arena of mutuality. The trajectory from object relating to usage (Winnicott, 1971) is reflected in the shift from mourning ritual to acts of commemoration that increasingly embody an intersubjective element. Those rituals move us out of grief's aloneness into a more complexly organized space that supports interior experience in an explicitly relational context.

*Yizkor* echoes this duality. On one level, we're alone with personal memories and grief during *yizkor;* no one moves to comfort others. Yet we also stand, speak, and sing together. I'm sometimes acutely aware of others' pains—of a friend who lost her husband when her children were small; another whose loss is fresher than mine. I'm among a temporary community of mourners; that awareness holds me without negating or minimizing my own losses.

The tension between the interior and intersubjective is embodied in many memorial rituals. While *yizkor* begins with individual prayers, the interior becomes communal when the group collectively recites *kaddish* and sings a communal psalm. As we sing together, we co-create a group of like mourners who function for one another as holding object, witness, and, of course, participant (Hagman, 1996, 2016; Orfanos, 1997, 1999; Solomon, 1995).

Whatever their shape, the dynamics of deep attachments are layered and complex. Our personal memorial stories exist at some distance from "truth"; they represent a more cohesive, emotionally meaningful, and consistent vision of our love objects—our ongoing relationship to, and separateness from, them.

Over time, we continue to memorialize, but this process isn't static; the emotional point of entrée for commemorative ritual is altered by new losses, a growing awareness of our mortality and our shifting dynamics. Since I began saying *yizkor*, I've confronted my own aging, experienced other losses and other joys. My first grandchild, Harry, was named after my father; my fourth, Eitan, after my mother. They have made my parents come alive again in a different way. I've also become far more able to imagine my way into my parents' responses to me and find it easier to identify with aspects of their own experience. Yet at the same time, my parents seem far more remote than in earlier years. I rarely think or speak about the world of my childhood; I've left that part of life, along with analysis, behind.

Still, when a major family event takes place, as when I lost a dear friend, earlier losses reemerge, reminding me that I'm at once connected to—and separate from—my parents. *Yizkor* offers me a fixed door through which to remember, to find what's lost but not forgotten.

## Memorials outside commemorative space

Acts of memorial take a wide range of forms. Memoir writing, for example, represents an explicit attempt to revisit the past and potentially to honor loved ones.

Which brings me back to the consulting room. For there's almost always loss inherent in an analytic relationship. While these connections are as intimate as any in our lives, they ordinarily end artificially rather than with actual death (except when they continue; Chapter 8). Certainly, termination helps us say goodbye, but once our goodbyes are said, neither analyst nor patient has easy ways of marking, much less memorializing, their relationship. Do these endings, sometimes quite stark and final, require their own memorial acts?

I wonder whether professional writing and speaking function—on a more procedural than conscious level—as symbolic acts of memorial. By writing about our patient or analyst, we evoke and rework that relationship, and, to some extent, memorialize it. In the process, we may also repair it. If we can and if we dare.

In his brief 1915 essay "On Transience," Freud described how the evanescent nature of beauty and love can block pleasure. He linked that difficulty to a "revolt in their minds against mourning" (p. 306). Freud noted that the price to be paid for avoiding the pain of loss is, paradoxically, a diminution of pleasure. It is as if the person says, "I won't love what I can't have, what won't last forever. If I love, I'll have to lose. So I won't."

Our phobic response to death has become, to some extent, culturally embedded. We avoid acts of commemorative ritual to let sleeping dogs (people) lie, to keep an emotional lid on distress. This dynamic emerges noisily in work around schizoid detachment but can infiltrate, even dominate, our response to traumatic loss. Those losses (especially early losses) aren't always remembered, much less fully mourned, because dissociation shuts down affect and forecloses engagement with memory.

My great-grandfather's sudden (and violent) suicide in 1929 (precipitated by the stock market crash) was a trauma the family couldn't encompass. My grandmother sent her children away without saying a word about why; they only learned about their father's death weeks later, from a neighbor's son. My mother wasn't taken to her father's funeral, no one sat *shiva*; indeed, his name was never again mentioned. And so, the family carried on, his death neither mourned nor communally remembered. There were no family stories about Grandpa Louis, no reminiscences, and no holding. When my maternal grandmother died decades later, this avoidant dynamic resurfaced: My mother, terrified of entering the arena of loss, begged the rabbi to conduct the funeral without having her go to the cemetery. Determined to remain upbeat and solid, she couldn't grieve and couldn't remember. For my mother, acts of memorial threatened to disrupt a fragile overlay that covered traumatic loss. It's not surprising, perhaps, that I've carried the desire to remember for us both.

For some, the defense against loss and grief is impenetrable. Susan, now 68, has a history of early trauma and dislocation. She's phobic about illness and death and cannot sustain even a nostalgic connection to her parents, long deceased. When her mother died (Susan was in her late 20s), Susan threw out everything belonging to her mother. Refusing to visit her parents' graves or even talk about her parents, Susan maintains some degree of emotional equilibrium by sealing off memory space. But her avoidance also infiltrates the present. Susan's adult sons wonder about the complete absence of any family stories; they've grown up as a solitary generation. More problematic, Susan can't be empathic when her friends are ill, can't tolerate anxiety or loss even at a distance.

There's an obverse, equally problematic edge to this dynamic: Addiction to loss and memorial ritual. When we remain absolutely embedded, "unseparated" from lost love objects, remembrance of things past interferes with our ability to embrace the present (this melancholic position stimulated the psychoanalytic emphasis on decathexis and working through). When Christie's 55-year-old brother died of heart disease, she was bereft. While Christie's grief seemed understandable to her family at the time, a decade later, their empathy has attenuated. Surrounding herself with mementos of Jonathan's life, reading the books he loved, Christie withdraws into her bedroom, detached from family life. Her grief is frozen and overwhelming; it blocks her reentry into the quotidian. Christie resists therapy and rebuffs her family's attempts to reach her. Christie has no access to a transitional realm that would help her move in and out of the experience of absence; she's as stuck in mourning as Susan is in denial.

It's unsurprising that many flee from the kind of experience in which Christie is submerged. We need to believe in the future, to embrace hope, and focusing on our history can feel like a counterweight to optimism. Yet at their best, memorial rituals allow us to access a transitional space that makes room for both connection and separateness, for merger and isolation (Winnicott, 1951). We don't challenge the "reality" of our loved one's simultaneous absence and presence just as we don't challenge the actuality of the analytic relationship.

## Beyond separation

Commemorative ritual not only counters the illusion of separateness, it preserves a continuity of experience that coexists with a sense of ourselves apart from our losses (Levi-Strauss, 1985). It helps us to reshape, even recreate aspects of a lost relationship within a communal holding space. Rather than choosing between renunciation and denial, we face our losses *and* affirm their aliveness within us. Both mourning and memorial ritual— illustrated here by *shiva* and *yizkor* tradition—represent a brilliant pre-psychoanalytic response to a universal human need. It's time we reject the psychoanalytic idealization of renunciation and separation and embrace our need to celebrate our capacity for connection.

## Postscript

My papers on mourning—mostly written in the early 1990s—were met with dozens of letters from colleagues (handwritten letters in those pre-email days) thanking me for reconnecting them to their own loss experience. While many wrote specifically about *shiva*, I also received letters from non-Jews who resonated with the process as it unfolded in their own cultural milieus. In my entire professional career, I have never received another such outpouring of personal letters. Clearly the need for holding exists across the lifespan for all of us, even for us "well-analyzed" analysts.

In memory of my father, Harry Slochower, my mother, Muriel Zimmerman, and my maternal grandmother, Belle Zimmerman. With deep gratitude to Minyan M'at, Sharon Penkower Kaplan, and my children, Jesse, Alison, and Avi.

Chapter 11

# The absent witness

## Mourning, virtually

What happens when we face massive losses but cannot access community? *Can* we mourn when even in 2023 we're at best semi-post-Covid? Do we analysts have the requisite psychic and reflective space to help our patients with something that continues to upend the quotidian for all of us?

Twenty-two months of horror dramatically undermined our ability to hold onto a necessary illusion—that, in Winnicott's terms, we could count on the world going on being. Not for the first time in history, to be sure, but for the first time in the lives of many of us. And the trauma we're contending with goes beyond Covid. Political crises, social upheaval, climate disasters, and wars all coexist with grinding absences. In the United States and elsewhere, we regularly witness incidents of appalling indifference and intentional destructiveness toward the Other. Widespread poverty and hunger, racially based police brutality, lack of access to vaccines and/or good medical care threaten us all. To make matters worse, democratic process is under direct attack worldwide[1]. Although each of us is differently activated depending on our personal circumstances, politics, and identifications, we've all been forced to contend with a mixture of grief, frustration, and rage.

To make matters worse, fissures between us have deepened. Antisemitism, Islamophobia, racism, anti-LGBTQ sentiment—to name a few—proliferate. The Other, a potential witness to our loss, may turn

---

1 The day before Putin invaded Ukraine, I was teaching therapists in Kyiv via Zoom. I was asked not to discuss the Russian invasion for fear of stirring intragroup conflict. But as the class ended, I found myself in tears and gave voice to the existential threat facing my colleagues and their country. Many met me with tears of their own. Only days later, they were hiding out in subway stations and treating their patients for free, remotely. Protected no more. My deepest respect and gratitude to my colleague Alyona Esse-Chukanova, who helps us all hold onto hope.

DOI: 10.4324/9781032691534-17

out to be an anti-vaxxer, a climate-change denier, an unapologetic racist. Someone in my own family, a Democrat-turned-Trumper, refused get vaccinated or even tested before visiting his grandkids. Concern for those he loves was superseded by politics. I find it impossible to feel empathy for those who—like him—refuse vaccinations even though doing so puts others at risk. And when the unvaccinated become ill, part of me feels they've gotten what they deserve. Have I, have we, become another version of Gerson's (2009) "dead third"? Can we act as witnesses only for those who reside within our own sociopolitical bubble?

We haven't all been equally affected by Covid. What Fors (2018) calls a complex power asymmetry allowed the privileged to limit exposure to the virus, gain access to vaccines and good medical care, and protect themselves from a myriad of other dangers. Some worked from home, retreated to weekend places, to family. Yes, there were limits even for the privileged; no one was entirely protected from illness or the multitude of other potential disasters we fear. But privilege determines how we live and, too often, *who* lives.

Even this "new normal" has been anything but constant. The arrival of the vaccine at the end of 2020, in tandem with Trump's defeat, fleetingly replaced helplessness and terror with hope. There were moments of near-manic relief; we could safely be together—hug, gather for holidays. But the arrival of new variants pierced that joy and demonstrated the limits of our capacity to remain protected. On one level, our pre-Delta/Omicron euphoria represented a necessary reaffirmation of the possibility that the future would eventually be better. On another, it demonstrated an excess of optimism that bordered on denial.

January 2023. We are in a different place—and not. The belief that the pandemic is nearly over, that the vaccine has saved us, has been repeatedly pierced. While Covid remains a distant threat, many have "gotten over" the pandemic; they've abandoned masks and treat the virus as a nuisance more than a risk[2,3]. Is this a realistic assessment of where we are now, or a manic defense? How careful *do* we need to be?

Our risk assessments always reflected our personal urgencies. To join a gathering of quadruple-vaccinated friends or err on the side of prudence

2 A recent article in the Guardian (3/13/2022) notes that "America's rush to normalcy has robbed us of the time to grieve our Covid dead."
3 See also Engels's (2022) essay on obstacles to mourning during Covid.

and stay home? Fly to see parents, grandparents, children, grandchildren? Work in person or remotely? Few of us were consistent. We played some degree of Russian roulette with Covid risk, the odds shaped by the urgency of our desires and our risk tolerance.

Through most of the pandemic I worked virtually and avoided indoor dining. Yet I repeatedly flew long distances to see my grandchildren because their absence had become intolerable. By contrast, one of my colleagues still won't get on a plane to visit family but meets his patients in his office, unmasked, reasoning that too much is lost when working virtually. I think that in both cases, we're less incautious than selectively, calculatedly cautious as we attempt to balance our needs and fears.

Omicron precipitated a PTSD trauma state in many of us because it reevoked the terror of March 2020. What we had counted on (that this is ending, that the vaccines would protect us fully) cannot be assumed after all. Will we who are older live out our lives forever wary of exposure?

Certainly, life's finitude confronted us even when Covid didn't threaten. Some of us are better at excluding or dissociating what can't be helped than others. But even those who ordinarily manage to sideline what derails may be especially strained right now. Because, even as the threat of Covid attenuates, we confront multiple dangers, including (but not limited to) Putin's invasion of Ukraine, Afghanistan's assault on women's rights, another onslaught of police attacks on African Americans and trans individuals, the continuing slaughter of American schoolchildren, climate disasters the Israel-Gaza conflict. I could go on.

Are we, as a song of my adolescence warned, on the eve of destruction? Can these devastating losses be mourned?

Some of us, of course, have done more than mourn; we've organized. We've pushed back against racist police brutality, cheered our healthcare workers, helped asylum seekers, offered treatment and immigration assistance to refugees, worked for climate change, political and police reform. Action is energizing; it moves us out of helplessness and toward agency. Embodied in activism is a form of enacted witnessing that can empower and strengthen our bonds to the Other and to our own communities.

## What we've lost

The ordinary. The illusion that the world will be all right despite period disruptions. To some extent, technology has stepped into the breach by allowing us to "be" with others virtually.

My patient Tania lost her mother to Covid in 2020. Tania was able to cry "with" me (on Zoom) in the days preceding her mother's death. It felt good, she said, to know I was there and that I cared. But she needed something more and held a Zoom wake, hoping to find comfort in the experience of being with friends and family—albeit on a screen (Trub, 2021; Trub & Magaldi, 2017). It didn't work; Tania found the wake anything but comforting and described how acutely "un-held" she felt as she stared at 75 tiles on a computer screen. This Zoom wake didn't facilitate a mourning process—if anything, it underscored her isolation. Tania said the following:

> As you know, I'm usually pretty good at expressing my feelings so it's totally weird to say this, but I can't really feel anything. It's like I'm shell-shocked. It's so different from when my dad died 10 years ago. Then, all my friends and relatives came to the wake. We sat around, ate, cried, hugged. It was incredibly reparative. Now, I'm all by myself. I want to cry, want to remember her, and say so many things to her and about her, but I can't. All I feel is aloneness and flatness. When people phone me, I go on automatic pilot, I thank them for calling, say a bit about my mom. But it's performative because I'm not really there. I can't feel them. It's like I'm half dead.

My ordinarily emotional patient found the virtual wake alienating; it left her feeling acutely and painfully isolated. I'm hopeful that in time she'll refind her feelings and that I'll be able to help her mourn. But not yet. Covid—really the restrictions it imposed—utterly blocked this for her.

Ironically, a friend of Tania's attended her Zoom wake and told her how wonderful he felt it was. He was moved by what was said and by his ability to see the faces of the mourners up close, on-screen. He could bridge the gap between the virtual and the actual in a way that Tania (the mourner) was not. After all, he wasn't in need of witnessing.

For those of us acting as witnesses rather than mourners, then, virtual memorial events can intensify our experience; faces and voices are up close, personal. We don't miss a word or expression and may be able to imagine ourselves part of a larger community of mourners and feel sustained. But these events are likely to be assimilated quite differently by the mourners themselves, depending, again, on their response to the absent in-person element.

As the Covid threat diminished, we gradually began to come together, to attend small in-person funerals, wakes, *shivas*, and the like. For some this has been a great help. In summer, a friend who lost a parent arranged for an outdoor *shiva* in a New York City park. People sat in socially distanced chairs and offered their condolences. We spoke later and she told me the following:

> ... I remain amazed at the difference between my Zoom *shiva*, in which I felt like I had to perform and was being looked at, and the comfort I felt when people showed up in person, the simple fact of being with them. Of course, being masked is not what I had hoped for, but still, despite that, it was a supportive, nurturing experience.

There's both loss and hope embedded here. Loss insofar as both the virtual and small in-person *shiva* fall so short of the ideal. Our inability to read social cues on large Zoom calls makes it near impossible to enter a conversation without risking cutting someone else off, or of several people speaking simultaneously. And, of course, the absence of eye contact bleaches the mourning experience of what is, perhaps, its most powerful element. Both Tania and my friend felt alienated by the virtual memorial events. Yet despite its limitations, the small, masked, in-person *shiva* provided what the virtual could not—embodied contact and a sense of being held.

The mourning experience always depends, of course, on the nature of our relationship to the lost Other, the number and kind of losses we carry with us, the presence or absence of other supports in our lives, and our personal trauma history. Those for whom current trauma recapitulates earlier losses will inevitably have more difficulty remaining in a protected mourning space than those for whom the present doesn't carry powerful emotional ghosts.

I'm referring both to our patients and ourselves. At times, we analysts may also become too flooded, activated, or preoccupied to be fully present for our patients. How to bracket our grief when it threatens to foreclose patients' access to interior process? Will we become crushed by our impotence, inured to grief, or carried away by our curative fantasies? After all, the mourning process requires sturdy witnesses. And we analysts aren't always that sturdy.

## When the analyst is also a mourner

When it's our own patient who dies—whether of Covid or something else—we confront a different emotional dilemma. Buechler (2000) and Frommer (2014) eloquently describe how the analyst's capacity to "be" with a dying patient can soften and ease the patient's experience. But for an analyst, the death of a patient creates a void. We become what Aronson (2009) calls the "undesignated mourner" (p. 255)—unrecognized and un-held. Who will help us mourn? Buechler (2000) notes,

> We have no institutionalized rituals for dealing with these losses. It is as though the fact that the person was a "patient" makes a ritual unnecessary. We would be unlikely, if a colleague, or friend, or relative died or permanently left, to expect ourselves to "move on" without grieving. But because, in some fundamental sense, our role encourages the denial of the personal impact of our relationships with patients, we also deny the personal meaning of their death or departure.
>
> (p. 84)

Here, then, is another way in which we can fail to make room for ourselves and our own sense of loss. Because our vulnerability exists *not* in tension with our analytic capacity, but instead as an aspect of it. To allow ourselves to mourn a patient's death without disrupting our sense of the professional requires that we encompass our vulnerability within our analytic identity.

Certainly, it's easier for us when it's our patient who needs to grieve. Whether we help someone mourn a death, a lost opportunity, the road not taken, or a decimated world, processing loss is a central aspect of the work we're trained to do. This is especially so when a patient's loss is covered by—or layered with—dynamic conflict or other unconscious issues.

But when loss creates a new existential reality—and particularly when we share that reality—we may be far less able to help. What can I offer a patient whose whole family contracted Covid at a cautiously planned, masked, outdoor wedding? Someone in despair as the business he built from nothing collapses? Or a person of color flooded with rage-infused grief at the indifference of his White coworkers to the deaths in his community? These kinds of existential realities assault our sense of going on being and threaten our capacity to remain emotionally responsive. Only if we can recognize, witness, and hold without denying our own grief can we help our patients mourn the multiple losses, personal and global, that they—and we—confront. But no matter how skilled and resilient we are, we're contending with individual and collective trauma that sometimes exceeds the clinical power of the work we do. There's simply too much traumatic loss.

It's my hope that we—and our patients—will find another path to grieving via our participation in commemorative rituals enacted over time (Chapter 10). Memorial rituals deepen our sense of being with our lost loved one *and* with others who also grieve. They may provide the very grounding sense of connection that's elusive right now.

Can this hold true when that connection is virtual? In January 2021, President Biden established a temporary memorial space for the 400,000 then lost to Covid. Candles were lit around the reflecting pool in Washington, D.C., followed by 400 bell tolls. Watching the ceremony on television, I found myself sobbing, briefly freed to grieve in the presence of an invisible virtual community. But then, I was not mourning a loved one, "merely" the loss of the world as I knew it.

In doing analytic work that doesn't negate the actual, we engage in a kind of activism that can stabilize and sustain us in the presence of so much that derails. We refind our capacity to offer something palpable to the Other. But we also need to make peace with the fact that our ability to help our patients mourn has its limits because the constraints we face aren't going away anytime soon. I refer both to the constraints imposed by Zoom and by the multiple realities that have destabilized our world—and us. It's precisely here that commemorative ritual may add a much-needed element. It can create a sense of collective, mutual holding, something we've been very much lacking.

We have to, I think, encompass a double reality: That we have much to offer our patients—and very little. That some of us have the emotional resources to open therapeutic space despite our vulnerability and some of us do not. While our personal need to mourn and commemorate may limit, if not foreclose, our capacity to be there for our patients, that shared vulnerability also can deepen our connections and enrich the work.

We need to help our patients—and ourselves—accept a new reality, one that has shattered so many illusions; that shakes, if not dismantles, the background assumptions about the world that we've relied upon. If we're to open reflective space and deepen our work despite those limitations, we need to acknowledge—but not become immobilized by—the grief dominating our world. To use analytic space to witness our patients' experience while simultaneously acknowledging the limits of that capacity.

# Chapter 12

# Factions are back

Psychoanalytic factionalism is alive and well in 2023. As old a phenomenon as psychoanalysis itself, our field's splits have shifted in content and varied in intensity but remain pressing and present. And while these splits mostly coalesce around ideas (both psychoanalytic and sociopolitical), there's nothing theoretical about them; they were—and are—deeply personal. Even as I worked on this chapter, painful new fractures have erupted in the field.

While we aim to help our patients tolerate ambiguity and move toward intersubjective exchange, we've had enormous difficulty doing this among ourselves. Here, I describe my personal encounters with psychoanalytic tensions and theorize their underlying dynamics. I hope it's not naïve to imagine that, were we to embrace an overarching psychoanalytic identification, we might begin to move toward open, thoughtful engagement and away from factionalism.

## Psychoanalytic training in wartime

When I was in analytic training at NYU Postdoc in the 1980s, there were two dominant tracks (the relational track didn't come into being until after I had graduated, and the independent track was pretty quiet during those years). The two active orientations, Freudian and interpersonal, were at war—well, at cold war. Candidates were sometimes recruited by competing tracks and pressured to choose, even though *not choosing* was explicit policy.

The caricatures were consistent—and consistently unfriendly: Freudians were rigid and unempathic; interpersonalists made superficial and/or undisciplined use of their countertransference while ignoring the patient's underlying dynamic issues. When they were even included in the conversation, self

DOI: 10.4324/9781032691534-18

psychologists were described as avoidant of conflict and inauthentically empathic. The notion that each had a contribution to make and that something good might accrue from cross-theoretical exchange was quite remote. Suspicious, both of alternate perspectives *and* of the analysts who identify with them, our theory—whatever its particulars—became part of our character armor (Reich, 1975).

It could have been worse. Like other training programs teaching multiple orientations, NYU Postdoc allowed (and both allows and encourages) candidates to take courses and get supervision in every track. Nevertheless, the implicit demand to take a side subtly affected many of us, albeit in variegated ways.

Across our institutes, these schisms have had a troubling impact on the way we train candidates. As Kernberg noted (1986, 1996, 2000), psychoanalytic education is frequently conducted in an "atmosphere of indoctrination" (1986, p. 799) that destroys candidates' creativity. Until recently, courses on comparative models were used largely as a vehicle through which to disparage the theory that wasn't the instructor's own. Rather than inviting candidates to query *all* perspectives and identify areas of overlap and difference between them, we taught them to pledge allegiance. To our flag. This despite Wallerstein's (1990) plea that we find the common ground among psychoanalytic theories.

I recognize that this piece of our history may come as an unpleasant surprise to current candidates in training and perhaps also to more recent graduates. This isn't the professional world most of you encountered (thank goodness). But it's a part of our history, and one worth remembering, particularly because it's the backdrop to the contemporary schisms that threaten us.

Inter-track conflicts at NYU Postdoc intensified further when a relational track was proposed in the late 1980s. Some interpersonalists felt that the relational movement was ignoring the significant overlaps between it and interpersonal theory (I think we were); others joined the relational track. These splits carried profound emotional meaning and took a personal toll on many of us (Kuchuck, 2013). Resultant feelings of betrayal and abandonment created what Kirsner (1990) described as siege mentality.

It turned out that our conflicts were a very mild version of the wider theoretical tribalism—often the wars—that dominated the American psychoanalytic field during those years. Each orientation was convinced theirs was the best; the others were to be ignored, scorned, sometimes despised. Too often that "other" theory came to represent the church, mosque, or synagogue to which one did *not* belong; as such, it represented a significant threat. Intertheoretical conferences were rare; when they did occur, they tended to devolve into ad hominem attacks, both of divergent ideas and of the person who thought and practiced differently. We candidates were both disturbed and puzzled by all this.

Equally troubling were the battles for dominance among American institutes. For example, the American Psychoanalytic refused to train "lay" (nonmedical) candidates, thereby protecting their financial fiefdom. Non-MDs were second-class psychoanalytic citizens. As, of course, were MSWs.

## Our theoretical schisms

The pressure to conform to a group's belief system (referred to as groupthink by social psychologists: e.g., Janis, 1972) was powerful. Our splits have haunted the field (Grand & Salberg, 2017; Kalb, in press). They've been a ghost that created hostile tribes and in- and out-groups, rather like religious institutions (Sorenson, 2000). Worse still, they rendered "new" ideas dangerous, whether those ideas grew out of the work of someone within a group or were introduced from the outside. When we did align with another orientation, it was usually against a third. It all reminded me of the Tom Lehrer 1965 song "National Brotherhood Week." I quote a stanza (and include a link):

> Oh, the Protestants hate the Catholics
> And the Catholics hate the Protestants
> And the Hindus hate the Muslims
> And everybody hates the Jews
>
> www.youtube.com/watch?v=allJ8ZCs4jY

Who the "Jews" were, of course, varied, depending on the alternate theory's preferences and biases (note that in other verses, Lehrer points to racial and socioeconomic divides; religion was/is only one of many such schisms).

The desire for uniqueness has led us to overemphasize difference, ignore theoretical overlaps, and caricature the other position. For decades,

American Freudians hated the interpersonalists who hated object relations and self psychology folk, and vice versa. In the eastern United States, nearly everyone hated the Kleinians and Lacanians. In California, where Bion and Klein have had more influence, and in Chicago, where self psychology pushed back against ego psychology, the groupings were a bit different. I'm not sure, though, that they were any less virulent. The notion that we could learn from the other theory or that cross-theoretical dialogue would enrich our thinking and clinical work collided with the need to prove that our theory was the best; indeed, the only good way to conceptualize psychodynamics.

Despite some exceptions (I think particularly of Loewald, who brought both ego psychological and interpersonal training to his brand of Freudian theorizing), we've mostly retained a reflexively suspicious, rejecting attitude toward the theory (or theories) with which we don't identify. We've had enormous difficulty moving toward what Willock (2007) called an integrative psychoanalysis that encompasses the schools of earlier decades (see also Kuriloff, 2010). Incidentally, for the lay public, our intra-psychoanalytic arguing has been both mystifying and alienating. Certainly, very bad for the profession overall.

## The theoretical is quite personal

Far more than theory drives our professional identifications and disidentifications. We learn in a relational context—from our teachers, supervisors, and, especially, our analyst(s). Yes, we also read. Our reading deepens, challenges, and expands our thinking, but it rarely shifts our professional identity on its own; conscious and unconscious dynamics play at least as large a part.

Our identifications are often informed, then, by the desire (not entirely conscious) to please those we idealize, to belong to a cohesive group, to garner approval from those we admire. We're pulled toward the position of our group, mentors, and/or analyst(s). For some, *not* aligning with the dominant theory evokes worries about losing collegial and friendship connections. Others try to demonstrate their independence from the powers that be by joining a splinter group.

To further complicate things, our chosen theory may represent a symbolic solution to our struggles or anxieties. I illustrate all this with a personal example and consider how those identifications do—and don't—reflect our work in the clinical moment.

My exposure to psychoanalytic thinking began well before I started training; my parents were both Freudian analysts and my identification with them, of course, informed my choice of profession. But when I entered graduate school, I encountered divergent perspectives that enriched my understanding and helped me begin to develop clinical skill.

Mainly, I discovered the object relations movement. Their focus on early, two body relationships was compelling. Winnicott's maternal, idealized perspective on both clinical work and maternal care especially spoke to me. Concepts like the holding environment, transitionality, and good enough mothering, in tandem with his normalization of hate in the countertransference, shifted my understanding of clinical process. They also helped me formulate the way I hoped to parent (*and* the ways I wished I had been parented).

Early in graduate school, I went into analysis with someone recommended by a beloved supervisor. My analyst self-identified as object relational and I responded to her empathy with relief; she offered me something very different from the rigid stance I had encountered in an early therapy experience and, later, in supervision with a classical Freudian.

But conflict was also embedded in this choice. My parents viewed my analysis with skepticism; my mother's mild question about whether the treatment went "deep" annoyed me, yet also evoked doubt. I wasn't altogether sure whether my choice of analyst was legitimate or a form of adolescent rebellion. *Was* my analysis superficial? *Should* I have sought out classical training?

Today, I think all the above: My Winnicottian identification, in tandem with my choice of analyst, partly emerged out of my intellectual and clinical sensibility. In the late 1970s, Winnicott's perspective seemed fresh and human. It also spoke to me for emotional reasons. Those included some leftover (then unconscious) early needs and issues in tandem with my (quite conscious) wish to separate from my parents, to create a JND (just noticeable difference[1]) from them, a way of being both like them *and* different. I chose (their) psychoanalysis, and then made it my own by shifting to a different theoretical framework that allowed me to create a distinct professional idiom. On another level, my move toward object relations embodied an identification with my analyst.

---

1  JND is a concept from experimental psychology developed by Ernst Weber.

Over time, I became aware of some more complex and troubling aspects of my analysis. In retrospect, I think my analyst was avoidant of conflict between us. She didn't easily consider her own contribution to moments of impasse. Yes, I wanted to be like her in some ways—warm and empathic—but I also wanted to be more solidly boundaried (like my parents) *and* more open to addressing the reenacted element (like my interpersonal supervisors and colleagues). I thus partially disidentified with my analyst as I had with my parents to find my own way of working.

Wanting exposure to other approaches, I chose a training program with multiple tracks. At NYU Postdoc, my Freudian supervisors (Shirley Feltman and Bert Freedman) provided perceptive, if traditional, clinical perspectives. However, Shirley's insistence that I maintain absolute boundaries with my first analytic patient blew that treatment up. I had sensed that my patient needed a flexible frame because adherence to the rules was itself traumatizing for her and I tried to persuade Shirley of this. But she believed in a strict adherence to the frame ("either she's in analysis or she's not"). I argued to no avail; eventually I reluctantly complied (after all, I was a first-year candidate). My distress about Shirley's rigidity was undoubtedly intensified by some childhood experiences that were reactivated by her unbending stance. All this despite the ways that, on a personal level, we had a very warm relationship.

My analyst suggested that I next work with Larry Epstein, an interpersonalist influenced by Winnicott. Larry was a very different kind of supervisor; rather than telling me how to practice, he encouraged me to find my own way. Larry's interest in transference and countertransference hate was especially useful as I encountered patients recently released from the hospital.

## Our identifications and their underbelly

At NYU Postdoc, I sought out courses across the tracks. I wanted to understand what informed each theory and how it shaped the clinical encounter. But in some classes, it felt unsafe to query the instructor's theoretical orientation or explore the intersection and collision of different positions. The pressure to conform was very much in the air, felt by most of my classmates (even those without analyst parents!). There were clear, if unwritten, rules about engaging in cross-theoretical collaboration or speaking appreciatively about a different orientation's clinical position. I felt a bit like a closet Winnicottian when in supervision with a Freudian, and like a Freudian when working with an interpersonalist.

Anticipating—often correctly—that I'd be met with a censorious response, I sometimes avoided raising what might be controversial. Similar issues surfaced in supervision; one of my Freudian supervisors intimated that it would be a big mistake for me to work with an interpersonal supervisor; my interpersonal supervisor wondered aloud why on earth I would want to work with a Freudian.

The impact of all this extended beyond our classes. At least into the early 2000s, we rarely attended events sponsored by a different track or invited people from other orientations to speak at our track's colloquia or conferences. Yes, some of us socialized across tracks, but perhaps a bit like RBG and Scalia's friendship, we mostly avoided discussing psychoanalysis.

There were exceptions. Some candidates argued openly with instructors and some supervisors and instructors encouraged us to challenge the assumed, examine our theoretical assumptions, and use our intuition as we worked. But some did not.

It was in this rather tense context that the relational movement appeared on the scene. Emphasizing the clinical power of enactments, relationalists critiqued earlier (classical and object relations) models that seemed to elevate the analyst's wisdom and power while infantilizing the patient (what Mitchell, 1984, termed a "developmental tilt"). Adding to this was the feminist critique of traditional psychoanalysis for its negation of maternal and analytic subjectivity.

I found the relational perspective both intellectually exciting and clinically useful. I also suspect that my shift toward relational thinking represented a compromise—a way of both identifying *and* disidentifying with my parents' (and analyst's) perspective. On one level, this shift embodied Loewaldian parricide; on another, a move toward separation.

Identified with both relational/feminist and Winnicottian models, I was determined to bridge this divide, to find a way to include the Winnicottian trope within the relational canon. But the course I proposed, "noninterpretive dimensions of analytic work," was roundly rejected (a relational person said they "wouldn't touch it with a 10-foot pole"!). The idea that relational theory could include Winnicottian holding was virtually heretical.

Some years later, Emmanuel Ghent stepped down from teaching the Winnicott course at NYU Postdoc and I took it on. (Object relations theories were taught in the relational track, more as part of our historical legacy than as a useful clinical approach.) Interested in addressing its collision with relational theory, I reformulated the holding metaphor and addressed its intersubjective dimension and clinical application beyond the theme of dependence (Slochower, 1991, 1992, 1993, 1994, 1996a, 1996b, 1996c, 1999, 2004, 2006c, 2013c, 2014a, 2014b, 2014c, 2014d, 2017a). Initially, my attempts to encompass both themes were met with skepticism; holding, it was argued, meant holding back (Bass, 1996), even gaslighting the patient.

This personal narrative describes the impact of parental, Freudian, inter-personal, and object relations orientations on my training and post-training experience. It's not, by any means, a unique story; fellow candidates and, more recently, post-training colleagues describe similar responses.

Requiring that analysts pledge allegiance to a particular psychoanalytic brand collides with the very thing our professional ideal represents—a capacity to remain self-reflective and flexible. But to acknowledge that our position (whatever its particulars) might not be the last psychoanalytic word opens us up to attack.

On top of this, it's been all too tempting to ignore or deny our roots—to act as if we invented our brand of psychoanalysis out of whole cloth, as if we ourselves are impervious to influence (Bloom, 1997). Were what Freud (1929–1930) termed the "narcissism of small differences" (p. 305) driven, as he suggested, by underlying hostility or aggression? By insecurity about our distinctiveness? Probably by all of these. Anxiety about our uniqueness, creative potential, and therapeutic efficacy all fueled competition between institutes and between individuals. And, of course, some of our theoretical differences were large, not small.

In addition to our intellectual interests and in tandem with the dynamic factors described above, remaining loyal to a particular group has financial implications. We demonstrate our theoretical/clinical loyalty to maintain our referral sources. Most institutes still require that candidates seek out a train-ing analyst from its own faculty, thereby maintaining their steady income stream; that financial loyalty rarely ends with graduation. After all, if my clinical position isn't the best, why would you refer exclusively to me?

## And then there's what we actually do

Here's a paradox: Despite the power of our theoretical identifications, our ideological loyalty isn't always evident in the consulting room. Sandler

(1983) and McWilliams (2004) note that most analysts develop a clinical theory specific to a given treatment rather than to an overarching model. When we're working, we adapt to our patient's vulnerabilities and needs while ignoring (rather than engaging) the clash between that adaptation and our declared theory. We blend—even blur—our position in the best interest of our patient.

The space between the ideal and the actual (Slochower, 2006/2014)—often a rather large space—has existed since our earliest beginnings; our failure to examine that space creates a shared fantasy of clinical consistency and perpetuates a myth of theoretical purity. We foreclose self-examination *and* fail to integrate "new" ideas that collide with our chosen model.

I learned about this phenomenon early: When I was a young adolescent, my mother, self-defined as a classical Freudian, mentioned that she was helping a patient get a (then illegal) abortion. I was puzzled; even as a teenager I knew this wasn't permitted. When I inquired, she matter-of-factly answered, "Either we're in the business of helping people or we're not." Her words (and the principle they represent) remain with me.

My mother's deviation from her declared commitment to neutrality was far from unique. A few other examples: A friend's classical analyst made a call on her behalf to help her get a job (she got it); another analyst lent their patient money. Both patients were grateful; when they asked their analysts to explain why they had "broken the rules," however, the analysts remained silent. I suspect they couldn't find a way to justify or integrate their actions with their theory.

On one level, contradictions between our beliefs and the actuality of our clinical work are evidence of our humanity, our willingness to meet our patients where they are. We sometimes ignore or override therapeutic rules when they seem to contradict patient need. When we can acknowledge and explore the personal and enacted elements informing these moments of "rule breaking"—or our refusal to bend the rules—we deepen our clinical understanding and, hopefully, move the process forward. When, however, we foreclose self-examination and go full steam ahead without a pause, we abandon our professional ideal and allow self-interest and/or impulsivity to dominate.

Unmetabolized countertransference feelings, in tandem with mutual enactments, can precipitate us unthinkingly away from our theory. I wonder whether my mother's feminist identification overrode her commitment to an abstinent, inquiring treatment model. Did she consider the possibility that she was skipping over her patient's conflict about terminating the pregnancy and enacting a maternal role in unanalyzable ways? Similarly, when the classical analysts described above provided their patients with concrete help, were they motivated by caring and a wish to be helpful and/or offering their patients what they themselves would have wanted? Were they unable to think about their own motivations or simply unwilling to bring their subjectivity into the treatment space for theoretical reasons?

When our clinical work diverges from our theory or when "outsider" ideas interpenetrate, we tend to sidestep these discrepancies. And although emergent theory sometimes extends our thinking beyond the confines of our preferred model (Cooper, 2015), this clinical reality—while reassuring—is rarely acknowledged. It's not always easy to parse genuine analytic responsivity from countertransference acting out and/or a range of self-serving motives that pull us away from our theory.

"Do as I say and not as I do" is hardly an inspiring psychoanalytic aphorism. Why is it so difficult for us to encompass our inconsistencies and think about what drives them? While this is especially true of young analysts, even senior analysts can feel conflict and/or guilt about what they're doing that they shouldn't or about what they're *not* doing that they think they should. Does fear of condemnation pull us to ignore, even disavow, the space between our theory and clinical practice? Those wedded to a classical model may feel guilty or conflicted if they choose to "gratify" a patient; those interpersonally or relationally identified may feel similarly about remaining neutral and non-self-disclosing.

Awareness of our investment in being viewed in a particular way (by our patient or ourselves) can be so uncomfortable that it invites denial/disavowal. Ken Eisold (1994) suggests that these anxieties are inherent to psychoanalytic work because we have so few clinical signposts that provide certainty about our effectiveness (see also Jacobs, 1983). It's far easier to ignore the space between being (a particular kind of psychoanalyst) and the way we do psychoanalysis.

When I began serving as associate editor on psychoanalytic journals, I periodically encountered reviews that either rejected papers with a theoretical focus divergent from the journal's own or required that the writer "translate" their theory into the language of the journal's orientation. Reviewers (especially junior ones) critiqued submissions that failed to adhere to that journal's orientation even when its editorial policy did not. The need to declare allegiance, itself dynamically driven, appeared to inform at least some critiques.

Ironically, an intolerance for complexity likely underlies these splits. It obfuscates something we could be proud of—our capacity to meet our patient where she needs to find us. But to encompass this we would have to loosen, and be prepared to query *but not abandon*, our commitment to the theory we've embraced. As a field, we've failed to investigate this space as deeply as we might.

I'm aware I can deviate from my relational and Winnicottian identifications in both directions; I'm sometimes more boundaried *and* sometimes more self-disclosing than my professional ideal would prescribe. In earlier analytic years, I felt discomfort about both. While I sometimes sought consultation, I never was able to sustain the level of clinical consistency I thought I should.

With time, however, those conflicts have mostly dissolved. This doesn't mean I'm always clinically consistent, but instead that I'm less thrown when I'm not; I'm far more comfortable trusting my intuition and am less preoccupied with analytic "shoulds" and "should nots." As I've discussed elsewhere (Slochower, 2019), experience and aging can support an easier, more fluid relationship between theory and practice.

## Beyond NYU: The Balkanization of psychoanalysis

Psychoanalytic schisms were evident across the first half of my professional lifetime. When I was in training, there was red rope divider at the New York Psychoanalytic Institute. It separated members from nonmembers; we who were not members had to sit at the back of the hall[2]. Interestingly, many of us accepted this unquestioningly. This phenomenon was far from unique to American psychoanalysis; a PEP search for "factionalism" yielded 60 articles addressing the power of theoretical splits in and between institutes across the globe (see, e.g., Bose, 2003; Eisold, 1994, 1998; Kirsner, 1990; Wilson, 2020).

2 The American Psychoanalytic Association's refusal to allow MDs to apply for clinical training didn't change until a lawsuit forced it to. That refusal resulted in the formation of Division 39 and NYU Postdoc among other training institutes accepting non-MD analytic trainees. But the rift between MD and "lay" analysts persisted for decades.

Other examples: Only a decade ago, an NYU faculty person told me in confidence that he couldn't accept an invitation to join a committee from a different track because it would be seen as an act of betrayal by members of his own orientation. He feared that, were he to agree, he would be rejected by his track. True? Anxiety? Hard to say, but the threat of social/theoretical/ professional ostracism remained powerful, at least in the eyes of some.

Also, almost a decade ago, I presented a paper critiquing what I called "relational excess" at an interpersonal institute and encountered a rather stunningly hostile and personal attack by several senior faculty. One person said, and I quote, "What were you thinking by presenting your paper at this institute?" I suppose I wasn't. Or at least, that I was being naïve to anticipate that my colleagues would welcome theoretical critique. (Had I not been relatively senior at that point, I suspect I would have pulled back from engaging in critique altogether.)

I've seen these schisms play out at conferences in the United States, Israel, and Europe. I was once ragefully attacked by someone who, offended by my view on Winnicott, insisted that they knew the "true" Winnicott and that I was just plain wrong. I was bemused more than upset, but again, had I been a younger analyst, their hostile response might well have shut me down. I've seen similar frontal attacks leveled at colleagues who stepped beyond the dominant theoretical position (as defined by the in-group). I suspect that these attacks become most forceful when the presenter is perceived to be a defector from the in-group rather than an outsider.

Several of my European and Canadian colleagues believe these theoretical wars lasted longer in the United States than elsewhere. Winnicott certainly thought so: In 1968, following a presentation of "the use of an object" at the New York Psychoanalytic Society & Institute in which he was mercilessly attacked, he remarked that he now understood why America was in Vietnam (Goldman, 1993, p. 210). *Was* American psychoanalysis especially polarized, or did this phenomenon manifest differently—but equally intensely—in other countries? I'm not sure.

## Our psychoanalytic roots and their dynamics

This pressure to conform has its roots in our psychoanalytic beginnings. In 1912, following Freud's break with Jung, a secret committee was formed around him; it included Jones, Abraham, Ferenczi, Rank, Sachs, and Eitingon. Members were expected to pledge ideological loyalty to the group, which urgently needed to "prove" the scientific basis for psycho-analytic ideas, to establish their legitimacy in a skeptical and competitive professional world. When a member's position shifted, the new work had to be collectively approved prior to its publication.

Freud's investment in establishing and controlling the evolution of psy-choanalytic thinking was, of course, deeply personal. His difficulty engaging in open debate with alternate viewpoints was understandable, given his desire to establish the legitimacy of this "new science" and protect it from external critique.

Further intensifying the pressure on early psychoanalysis was the fact that this was a period of massive social, economic, and political upheaval. Conflicts between conservative and liberal factions in the 1920s Weimar Republic, in tandem with rampant antisemitism (Gay, 1968; Wilson, personal communication, 2023) confronted early psychoanalysts (mostly Jewish) with a fractured and terrifying world even before the Holocaust (see Prince, 2009; Young-Bruehl & Schwartz, 2012).

Freud likely established psychoanalytic training in free-standing insti-tutes outside the university system for several reasons: Both Austrian and German universities were deeply conservative and antisemitic, hardly an inviting home. Additionally, Freud was concerned that those unfamiliar with psychoanalytic thinking—i.e., university academics—would not be able to appropriately evaluate or respond to its complexities. But an unfor-tunate consequence of Freud's removal from academia was that American psychoanalysts were rarely trained in rigorous academic settings, gener-ally didn't learn to do research, engage in critical debate, or self-critique. Further, because psychoanalytic work is inevitably personal, neutral intel-lectual debates pose a particular difficulty for us (Joel Whitebook, personal communication, April 8, 2023): In many ways, that difficulty has followed us into the present day.

Prince (2009) and Young-Bruehl and Schwartz (2012) underscore the impact of psychoanalysis' trauma history on the splits that dominated the field. Because trauma blocks access to a mourning space and interferes with the establishment of collective memory, there was little space within which to encompass and process these splits, much less to move toward a more integrative and pluralistic way of conceptualizing.

Freud's death coincided with the beginning of the Second World War. The destruction of European Jewry, combined with the loss of home-land, disrupted personal and communal history. Emigration (for those

who were able) added to the trauma caused by the Holocaust. Jewish analysts fled the continent—to England, the United States, and South America.
But for many reasons, psychoanalysts didn't always find a welcoming
home in their new country—because they were lay, rather than medical
analysts (in the United States), in England because they weren't Kleinians
(T. Kohut, 2020) and/or because of the financial and interpersonal threat
they represented to local psychoanalysts. Thomas Kohut (2020) describes
his and his father's (Heinz's) experience of rejection at the hands of fellow psychoanalysts when Kohut's theorizing diverged from the dominant
ego psychological orientation of his colleagues (J. Anderson, personal
communication, April 8, 2023).

## A shift away from psychoanalytic factionalism?

It was imperceptible at first. But by the early 2000s things began to shift
away from the hostile intertheoretical fights of earlier years, at least
on the East Coast. We started talking to one another across the aisle
with less defensive self-protectiveness. And this has continued. Today,
many institutes offer at least one course in comparative theory; some
even invite "outsiders" to teach those courses. Course reading lists often
include essays from theories beyond the instructor's own. These comparative courses are far less reflexively condemnatory of the other theory
than they were. Some explicit attempts to engage in theoretical/clini-
cal *self*-critique and invite cross-theoretical dialogue have also appeared
(Aron, Grand & Slochower, 2018a, 2018b). At NYU Postdoc, inter-track
collaboration has become more the rule than the exception. There are
even beginning discussions of eliminating the track system. This would
have been blasphemy a decade ago.

Things have changed on a global level as well. Relationalists sit on
the editorial boards of *JAPA* and *IJP;* Freudians and Kleinians sit on the
board of *Dialogues* and other interpersonal journals. We teach at each
other's institutes, invite each other to speak at our conferences. Several
non-Freudian institutes in New York (including the WAW Society, Karen
Horney, and NYU Postdoc) were invited to join the American and IPA;
all voted to do so, something that would have been unthinkable even a
decade ago. Panels are rarely organized around proving that the alternate
theory is misguided; cross-fertilization is increasingly recognized and
valued.

An example: Today the notion of enactment, while defined somewhat differently depending on the analyst's orientation, is now widely accepted across theoretical divides. In part, this can be attributed to our easier access to multiple psychoanalytic perspectives. What's familiar is less threatening and we've had far more exposure to other ways of working in recent years. We've moved out of our theoretical cubbyholes, away from binaries, and toward a dialectic perspective on our own *and* the Other theory. All this has also been facilitated by technological advances—both the availability of online journals from different orientations and (a consequence of Covid) the possibility of attending virtual conferences across the theoretical and geographic world.

Beyond our theoretical expansion, we've become more inclusive of other clinical professions; many institutes now accept MSWs and other mental health practitioners for training where previously only Ph.D.s, PsyDs, and MDs could apply. Yes, in part this shift can be attributed to the organizations' financial need, but I think there's more to it; a recognition that otherness can be encompassed, that it's near impossible for any theory to entirely cocoon itself from others. Easier access to multiple points of view invites more cross-theoretical conversation; our "big theoretical tent" is far bigger than it was. And less divisive.

## Does pluralism have an underbelly?

Yes. There's an underbelly to every psychoanalytic position, including one that expands our borders and steps back from theoretical conflict. In the process of questioning our conviction that we've got the best theory, we lose a sense of certainty and, potentially, of intellectual self-confidence.

Further, identifying with a particular theory isn't inherently a bad thing. It supports the development of a professional identity, deepens our connection to like-minded clinicians, and provides an organizing function in the face of confusing clinical material. Giving up our "most favored theory" status weakens the power of our cohesive group; if we're no longer unique or entirely distinguishable from other models, it's possible an alternative perspective could offer something that we do not. Questions like "Might we be missing something?" engender self-doubt and may undermine our connection to our own theory *and* those who share it. After all, if your position is as valuable as mine, what's the point of remaining loyal, theoretically, clinically, or personally, to what was "ours"?

Further, too much blurring can obscure more than clarify. We run the risk of becoming so much of a "happy psychoanalytic family" that we sidestep or fail to engage our differences to avoid conflict. I'm thus decidedly *not* suggesting that we have moved—or should move—away from cross-theoretical critique. Our encounters with differing perspectives push us to examine, define, and refine our own vision of therapeutic action more sharply. We *need* both self-critique and critique from without, uncomfortable though the latter may feel. Lew Aron (2017) underscores precisely this in his essay "Beyond Tolerance." Describing the theoretical multiplicity characteristic of contemporary psychoanalysis, Aron notes that external critique invites us to "ambivalate" [*sic*] our own belief system—that is, to destabilize the assumptions on which we've unthinkingly relied. He invokes Benjamin's (1995a) ideas about rupture and repair to underscore the gains that can be derived from theoretical discord. Provided such arguments are lodged in a position of respect and recognition (something that cannot be taken for granted), they may help us move past polarization, deepen our thinking, and shift toward intersubjective dialogue. Arguing for what he calls "critical pluralism" and against the pressure to adhere to a given model, he[3] suggests that:

> getting along and mutual respect, peaceful coexistence, is not sufficient . . . Tolerance is essentially the granting of the right for the other to be mistaken, but not in any way a recognition of their viewpoint being of value.
>
> (p. 274)

Self-critique allows us to reexamine our belief system from the outside in, to destabilize the assumptions on which we've unthinkingly relied. When we engage with, rather than opposing or negating, theoretical/clinical differences, we're pushed to think harder, to define our own vision of therapeutic action more sharply. We're more likely to examine our blind spots.

Rather than aiming for a single "psychoanalytic demilitarized zone" then, cross-theoretical critique can be a powerful instrument of change. When

---

3  Aron (2017) suggests that on one level Freud himself was a reflexive skeptic.

we dialogue with difference from a position of mutual respect rather than defensive alienation, we open the door to recognition (Benjamin, 1995a) of the Other position; this in turn can help us find what binds us while addressing, rather than denying, the contradictions inherent in our own position. If the Other's contribution has the potential to be an asset more than a threat, we won't have to collapse what distinguishes us *or* attack the other theory for what it lacks.

Theoretical/clinical dialogue, then, can help us engage our thinking from the outside in and deepen our understanding of its value and limitations. We've begun to move this way and I see evidence of this shift at personal *and* institutional levels[4]. Might this shift signal the field's move toward a broader, overarching self-identification? After all, we're all analysts, we're committed to deepening our understanding of ourselves and the other. And we share a great deal despite what divides us.

## New sociocultural and psychoanalytic wars

I first drafted this essay in 2020, before these conflicts erupted. I titled it "Are We Nicer Now" because I thought we mostly were and sought to name and theorize why.

I was dead wrong.

Yes, our psychoanalytic wars are mostly over; we no longer attack one another for our theoretical beliefs. Thank goodness.

But. Where our earlier exchanges were organized around questions about the life of the mind, today, it's external, sociopolitical factors that dominate intellectual intercourse. Yes, psychoanalysis has always been impacted by sociopolitical events, but mostly outside—not inside—our profession. Today, though, those conflicts have penetrated our insularity.

---

4 Lest I overstate, it's worth nothing that elements of professional splitting lurk beneath these ideological détentes. We remain close to our theoretical homes when we write. While psychoanalysts across the continuum now cite the classic papers (e.g., Freud, Klein, Loewald, and Winnicott), it's less common for writers to reference contemporary papers on a chosen topic when those papers represent a divergent theoretical position. Yes, in part, these divides reflect our intellectual (and narcissistic) commitment to a particular point of view. But they also represent the residue of older theoretical battles, or at least, a need to honor their legacy.

To make matters worse, the tide has tilted sharply away from multi-culturalism and openness; conflicts around race, political affiliation, gender identity, climate change, Russia-Ukraine, and most volatile of all, the Israel-Palestinian conflict, play out beyond *and* within the field. Several issues have been particularly destabilizing. First was the Black Lives Matter movement (see, e.g., the documentary *Black Psychoanalysts Speak* (2014), Powell's essay (2018), and the Holmes Commission's (2023) report). The not-very-latent racism within psychoanalysis has surfaced; despite our avowed liberalism (Fors, 2019), the veneer of "niceness" we would like to call our own has mostly dissolved, revealing unmetabolized racially based hatred, contempt, and defensiveness among us.

In early 2023, a schism between pro- and anti-Zionist/Palestinian psychoanalysts added another dimension to these group conflicts. Initially triggered by public accusations of antisemitism leveled at Lara Sheehi, furious accusations and counterattacks erupted in many American psychoanalytic circles and played out on multiple listservs. Yes, there have also been efforts at genuine, respectful discourse, but they're dwarfed in impact, if not in number, by highly charged, accusatory listserv postings. Personal and professional relationships have been upended; group cohesion disrupted, and intersubjective recognition foreclosed. Some listservs were temporarily shut down in a (not very successful) attempt to contain the vitriol.

The October 7 Hamas attacks and Israel's response, in tandem with a global upsurge in antisemitism, have further intensified these splits. They override the many ways in which pro- and anti-Zionist Americans otherwise share similar politics and are often aligned (at least manifestly) against racism and other conservative policies.

Hatred of the other has once again invaded our no-longer-protected space. We may not hate one another for the way we do psychoanalysis, but we hate those whose beliefs clash with our own. There's something wearily familiar—and demoralizing—about our descent into name-calling and splitting.

I am no longer convinced that the world will move past the current crisis. As Grand (2023) notes, the paranoid schizoid position dominates. We seem unable to encompass our own history, identify our perpetrator parts, or allow ourselves to empathize with the rage of the suffering other. Grand argues that we need to recognize our own desire for vengeance and too-easy retreat to othering. To address our complex history as (often Jewish) victims of persecution *and* as White oppressors.

Certainly, our professional battles pale in comparison to the existential threats we face. But still. Our inability to engage with the Other position respectfully and reflectively is disturbing. Antisemitism, racial trauma, and the ongoing Israel-Palestinian conflict reactivate, even repeat, aspects of a PTSD trauma state for survivors and descendants of the Holocaust, the *Nakba*, and violent attacks on Palestinian and Jewish individuals world-wide. Are we frozen in a state of conflict because it embeds both personal and historical trauma?

To some extent, these schisms also embody a generational fracture—younger (Palestinian-identified) vs. older (Israel-identified) analysts. More than a few of my older colleagues have expressed the feeling that they've been rendered irrelevant by the actions and beliefs of the younger generation. Is there an element of symbolic parricide embedded here (Loewald, 1979)? Perhaps. But not more than an element; there are plenty of older and younger individuals on both sides of the issue.

I want to end this chapter on a hopeful note, to argue that these painful and destabilizing splits will give way to recognition of the Other's position and acceptance of difference. That we can reassert our humanity and capacity for empathy in a world more fractured and threatened than, perhaps, at any time since World War II. To do so, we need to override the splits and threats emanating from multiple sources, embrace what binds us (our psychoanalytic and citizen identifications), and find a way to hear each other across the political aisle as we have across the theoretical one. Must the repetition compulsion (whatever we call it) continue to hound us because we have not, in the end, sufficiently turned our psychoanalytic ghosts into ancestors? Is it too much to hope for civilized intellectual discourse lodged in positions of mutual respect? I fear this is wistful/wishful thinking.

I so hope not.

# Chapter 13

# Creating inner space
## The psychoanalytic writer

Professional writing came easy to me; that is, until I became a psychoanalyst. The emotional complexities of finding and sustaining one's psychoanalytic voice is the subject of this essay; a fitting way, I think, to end a book. I begin with my colleague Karen.

Karen opened our supervisory session by asking if I thought she was developed enough as a psychoanalyst to try her hand at writing. Her work with a very difficult and unusual patient had stimulated several ideas and she thought her perspective might be a new and interesting one. I agreed, and we began discussing her ideas in depth. Karen left the session feeling hopeful, planning to begin writing that very weekend. When she came in the following week, however, Karen was utterly deflated. On her own, facing the blank computer screen, she became intensely anxious and unable to proceed. With sudden clarity and utter certainty, Karen realized that her voice was inarticulate, "old hat," insufficiently incisive. Karen felt humiliated by the naïveté that had led her to think of writing. She had a chilling image of the amusement, derision, even wrath of certain senior analysts as they read her paper. How dare she tread where they dwelled? Even before beginning, Karen gave up.

Karen knew these anxieties well; she had dealt with them in analysis over many years. But despite considerable insight, Karen couldn't put her terrors aside and enter the arena of creative activity. The mere prospect of articulating her own voice raised the alarming specter of the Other. Creative desire collided with creative anxiety and resulted in inner collapse.

We take a leap of faith when we embark on a writing project. That leap, which coalesces differently as a function of who we are and the context (personal and professional) in which we write, inevitably involves subjective (and sometimes objective) risk. That psychoanalytic writing has its roots

DOI: 10.4324/9781032691534-19

in an academic tradition provides us with a layer of protection not afforded the creative artist. We write within defined parameters; there are sources to cite, models to follow. At the same time, our field allows us wide latitude within which to articulate our personal idiom; we aren't bound by the rules that govern much academic writing. But this creative space has its attendant risks. The aspiring psychoanalytic writer faces a daunting wealth of literature articulated from multiple theoretical and clinical perspectives. To construct or modify theory, to offer a new way of viewing clinical material, to integrate or criticize the work of others, all require that we take account of and respond to the work of others while also making an original contribution.

## Writing as a relational act

Like all forms of creative activity, psychoanalytic writing is both a solitary act and a form of communication to the Other. It serves a variety of functions for the individual writer. In the process of articulating our ideas, we may discover a new way to organize or integrate theoretical and clinical issues. Writing about patients can support—or alter—our treatment stance and deepen our understanding of our patient and ourselves. Since many of us write about areas of personal concern, we also can use writing to work indirectly on our own issues and/or communicate indirectly with our own (ex)-analysts.

But psychoanalytic writing is also exposing—of our patients and ourselves. What might we unwittingly reveal? Just how much of ourselves can we bear to make known (Grundy, 1993)? Will we be (mis)understood, recreated, even made over? The reader, a voice from "without" (Ogden, 1994), is likely to make over our text in line with her own perspective. In the process we risk being transformed, even negated. To manage the dialectical tension between recognition and nonrecognition inherent in being read, we must locate and sustain our own voice while enjoying, or at least tolerating, the inevitable misreadings that occur in communication between separate subjects.

In writing, then, we locate ourselves vis-à-vis other theoretical positions. Our hope that we have something new to say may evoke a simultaneous need to echo and rebut the position of our professional ideal. The "anxiety of influence" (Bloom, 1973) speaks to the concern that we haven't been as original as we had hoped. That anxiety can exert silent pressure on us to minimize our debt to professional predecessors—to creatively invent or misread the work of others in an unconscious attempt to bolster the uniqueness of our own contribution (Smith, 1997).

Psychoanalytic essays on the writing experience emphasize the dynamic meanings of writer's block (e.g., Bergler, 1955; Loewald, 1979). Writing can arouse an unconsciously wished-for and feared destruction of, or challenge to, the parental object or sibling. It can evoke the danger of negation in tandem with the paradoxical needs for recognition and privacy (Benjamin, 1998). Ultimately, we need to both contain *and* contend with self-doubt and anxiety, to sustain a personal voice without utterly excluding other thinkers' ideas.

## Our professional world

The contemporary psychoanalytic world is extraordinarily complex and theoretically diverse; it confronts us with the confusions and potential threats represented by multiplicity. To further complicate things, we write for professionals whose vocation involves exploring individual and interpersonal dynamics; there's a risk that we'll feel personally as well as professionally stung by critique. It's not necessarily paranoid to anticipate that both our text and personal dynamics will be scrutinized and misconstrued.

The anxieties associated with psychoanalytic writing will, of course, be intensified or diminished as a function of our vulnerability to criticism and judgment on one hand, and our capacity to enjoy intellectual engagement and challenge on the other. For some, writing evokes excitement, a sense of adventure, anticipation of a warm reception or even a good fight. We may enjoy the fantasy that our ideas are brilliant and will awe senior colleagues. But those visions may also evoke a fear of retaliation by those who have been "shown up."

Writers like Karen, however, become immobilized by the anticipation of failure and/or critique by the Other. Although new writers are especially vulnerable to these anxieties, some struggle with self-doubt across their careers; they worry about the value of their contribution and/or the consequences of success.

Carol, a prolific writer, described her writing process in the following way: When she becomes stalled, she reads the literature, which helps stimulate ideas and clarifies her own thought process. She reads freely and without anxiety. Yet Carol becomes terrified when facing the computer screen. She manages these anxieties by writing in total privacy, altogether avoiding the relational world until convinced that her work is perfectly sculpted and beyond reproach. Unable to imagine a benign response from the reader, Carol withdraws altogether from the relational arena to write. In so doing, she evades, rather than actively engaging, critique.

Carol's relational anxieties organize around the threat of annihilation. When she was a child, Carol's parents reacted to symbolic acts of assertion by attempting to subdue, retaliate, or demolish her voice (both verbally and physically). Their repeated rebuff of her spontaneous gesture (Winnicott, 1960b), now internalized, raises the stakes associated with the creative act (Barwick, 2000, 2003).

Other writers' anxieties are organized differently. While some fear the rejecting, punitive, or dismissive response of authority figures (e.g., journal reviewers, senior institute faculty, their analyst, etc.), others fear retaliation by symbolic siblings (colleagues or other professional competitors).

Ron harbored long-standing resentments toward some of his colleagues and mentors. Those resentments were based on both real experiences of rejection and his own competitive feelings. Ron needed to show his colleagues up, to prove he was right, that he knew better. When he came across a paper that seemed better than his, he fell into a state of despair, abandoned his efforts, and retreated (literally) to his bed. With encouragement from his analyst and friends, Ron eventually began writing again. However, his need to argue tended to flatten his work and render it one-dimensional. Ron couldn't stay with or play with his own ideas in a non-adversarial way.

Writers like Ron experience the outside world as dangerous; for them, the creative endeavor is fraught with risk. For others, the sense of threat is linked to the actual subject of the essay. Clinicians often are drawn to write about issues that have (indirect, if not explicit) personal meaning. Amir immigrated to the United States from the Middle East in early adolescence. For his Ph.D. thesis, he decided to write an essay about the psychological experience of immigration. Although he had previously written on more emotionally neutral topics without excessive struggle, Amir selected this topic in a quasi-conscious attempt to confront and rework his own immigration experience.

As the essay evolved, however, Amir became stalled, overwhelmed with anxiety. In an unconscious fantasy he eventually contacted, Amir stepped over his father's grave as he submitted the essay for publication. His father (who was still alive) had failed to learn English or in other ways acculturate. The subject matter of Amir's essay stimulated conflict around separation and oedipal issues that had not been previously evoked. Those issues effectively stopped Amir in his creative tracks.

## Writing and gender

Although men and women alike are vulnerable to the kinds of relational dangers I've described, feminist writers suggest that gender has a qualitatively different effect on women writers. Because the act of writing literally takes the mother from her child's side, creative expression collides with the mother's wish to meet the child's needs (Benjamin, 1995a; Deutsch, 1973; Lazarre, 1976; Suleiman, 1985).

How can the mother take on the reality of other separate perspectives, much less write about them, if she expects herself to focus only on the other? That focus narrows—even forecloses—the transitional space crucial to creative expression by blocking access to relational wishes. The prospect of "taking on" the other fails to bring about a competitive, quasi-erotic charge. Writing arouses not a desire to "fight back" or "penetrate" the other (Aron, 1995; Grundy, 1993) but, instead, a sense of defeat. Creative and relational desire collide and the writer collapses, unable to access her own idiom or play with the interface of her and others' ideas because writing symbolizes an abandonment of the relational world. While the germ of an idea may be toyed with, perhaps presented in a session or meeting, it quickly dissolves.

Other writers are more vulnerable to the immobilizing impact of self-doubt. Susi was so tormented by the fear that her ideas were insubstantial that she began and then abandoned essay after essay. Susi couldn't enter the realm of the imaginary, couldn't entertain creative fantasy, because she found it impossible to access and articulate ideas within the private space of her mind. Her profound self-doubt probably originated in childhood; although neither punitive nor retaliatory, Susi's parents were mostly absent emotionally (D. Stern, 1985; Stolorow and Atwood, 1992). She grew up without a solid capacity to articulate and sustain internal process, a capacity likely based on the mother's ability to contain the infant's mind

(Reiner & Bail, 1997). It was virtually impossible for Susi to tolerate the multiple "truths" that presented themselves when she confronted complex psychoanalytic issues.

These kinds of anxieties probably have more often plagued women than men. And, certainly, a baby represents an especially palpable inter-ference for the writer/mother. Nevertheless, I would reframe this dilemma in broader terms, for I don't believe it to be inherently gender related; the "female" and "male" represent alternating (and culture-bound) strains in all of us (e.g., Aron, 1995; Benjamin, 1995a; Dimen, 1991; Goldner, 1991; Harris, 1991).

Elsewhere, I've linked Winnicott's (1971) notions of "being" and "doing" to two different analytic functions while explicitly separating these func-tions from actual gender (Slochower, 1996a, 1996b). "Doing" describes the analyst's active, interpretive, relational, or boundary-setting functions, whereas "being" represents the analyst's aliveness and capacity to establish a private space for self-elaboration.[1] Winnicott contrasted the containing "being" function with "doing"; that is, with the active creation of a bridge to the world and implicitly to separateness. Although he didn't uniquely ascribe "being" to women and "doing" to men, he did connect the female/maternal element with the former and the male/paternal element with the latter[2] and underscored the prevalence of dissociative processes in single sex identity (which he believed contains an element of normal bisexuality).

## "Being," "doing," and creative process

"Being" and "doing" self-states provide a window through which anxious or conflicted writers can establish an insulated transitional holding space within which to create "new" psychoanalytic ideas. This protected space excludes core subjective threats to the writing process and shields the writer from debilitating self-doubt, thus helping the writer sustain a creative writ-ing space (Deri, 1976).

"Doing" anxieties are organized around the consequences of action. Writers plagued by these relational concerns fear the (real or internal)

---

1  See Bollas (1996) for a related discussion of these different analytic functions.
2  Benjamin (1995b) also criticized Winnicott's association of "being" with the female element and of "doing" with the male element.

reader's critical eye and the danger that they'll reject her work (Barwick, 2003). One response to "doing" anxieties is the evocation of antidotal fantasies that expand the writer's sense of power vis-à-vis the threatening reader or audience. These object-related fantasies, both oedipal/erotic and preoedipal, counter the vulnerability evoked by creative action. At the origin of such defensively organized self-states lie anxieties about one's potency and importance within an interpersonal context.

While struggling to write his first paper, Peter was preoccupied with the fear that his supervisor would rip his idea to shreds. After reading his supervisor's new paper, Peter excitedly described its serious theoretical flaws. Buoyed by the fantasy that he had surpassed this mentor/father and would receive the recognition for which he longed, Peter returned home and virtually dashed off his own paper. "Doing" fantasies helped Peter temporarily move past self-doubt; at the same time, they disrupted his connection to his supervisor and left him feeling both guilty and anxious.

At times, the experience of creative impotence has an erotic element. When the writer's ideas seem neither "big enough" nor "exciting enough," fantasies that reverse that fear can be engaged defensively. Like Peter, Nina imagines that colleagues will respond to her paper with enormous excitement, that she'll be both admired and (erotically) desired. Her antidotal fantasies allow her to write; the erotized relational threat is subjectively turned on its head: Her colleagues won't dismiss her; she'll excite them.

Writers who embrace illusions based on "doing" manage narcissistic vulnerability by actively taking on the other. The writer's primary identification is as actor; that is, as a subject residing in a world of other objects and subjects. Aron (1995) suggests that fantasies of grandiose (bisexual) omnipotence protect the writer from the fear of penetrating the intellectual arena in a state of sexual incompleteness. "Doing" anxieties are countered by "doing" fantasies: The writer imagines surpassing those who came before, even destroying or remaking the psychoanalytic world. Like the preoedipal child's identification with both parents in an overinclusive denial of sexual difference (Fast, 1984), these fantasies help the writer hold contrasting ideas in mind. A transitional space allows the writer to develop new ideas without making sense of them in ways that prematurely truncate creative process.

Omnipotent "doing" fantasies, then, represent an unconscious response to anxieties about action, about the consequences of penetrating the world of psychoanalytic theory in a state of incompleteness. As compensatory fantasies, they're empowering. On a more unconscious level, though, they leave underlying vulnerabilities reversed rather than engaged. They obscure, without resolving, the writer's self experience as the anxious child of professional parent(s). This manic (and implicitly defensive) phase of the creative process must thus be followed by a second phase in which the author subjects creative work to external evaluation.[3]

"Doing" anxieties and "doing" fantasies are lodged in the relational domain. They're less relevant to the writer who's struggling simply to remain "in her skin" and trust the potential value of her words. Writers like Karen cannot access and sustain their words at all; they never quite arrive at the point where relational anxieties are evoked. It's here that antidotal "being" self-state illusions may foster creative process where "doing" fantasies cannot.

It's paradoxical that retreating to an idealized "being" self-state can facilitate creative process. "Being" is ordinarily associated with containment and the inhibition of self-expression (Winnicott, 1971). The mother facilitates the baby's capacity for object relating because she doesn't require that the infant sort out the projected from the real aspects of her personhood; she contains her separate subjectivity. An identification with the "being" state could well create internal pressure *not* to delineate the edges of a separate voice.

Mary was working on a qualifying paper when she became preoccupied with the worry that an emergency was unfolding at home while she sat at the computer. Notably, she didn't feel this anxiety while seeing patients. We eventually came to understand that her anxiety was linked to an unconscious conviction that by retreating to her computer she was injuring her child; Mary imagined her little girl to be mournfully alone and bereft while she immersed herself in the rich world of ideas. Interestingly, that anxiety wasn't stimulated when Mary left her daughter to take on a caretaker position with patients.

But there's another side to these "being" anxieties. At times, invoking a maternal "being" illusion can erect an arena of creative certainty that excludes creative anxiety. This being illusion can represent a crucial layer

---

3 While the ego ideal can facilitate creative process (Eigen, 1993), idealization is more classically viewed as an interference in creative process because it interferes with a tolerance for imperfections (Freud, 1914).

of protection against paralyzing, hypercritical self-scrutiny. It supports an experience of interiority by temporarily excluding the threatening object world (Slochower, 1999, 2004, 2014c).

## The evolution of creative process: A personal journey

During the early years of my career, I worked in academic social and clinical psychology where I wrote papers and a data-based book with comfort and ease. The format of that work was highly prescribed, its content tightly linked to research design and data analysis. Very little of "me" was expressed (or exposed) in my writing and the contents didn't carry symbolic meaning (other than as a means for gaining tenure).

But about 10 years in, my interest in empirical research waned and I turned to psychoanalysis. Lacking the format—and shield—of data-based research design and APA publication format, my writing felt "up close and personal"; it put me on the line in a very different way. Yes, I wanted to write, but I was overwhelmed with anxiety. Self-doubt collided with creative desire; I was more worried about the value of my ideas than related relational risks. Would I create a thin, insubstantial piece? Would my inadequacies be exposed? Would I inadvertently reveal something about myself that I was unaware of?

My anxieties, then, were lodged primarily in the "being" arena. They were debilitating. In fact, I didn't write at all until I had aired these feelings to a particularly responsive supervisor. He confidently confirmed the value of my ideas and offered to help me get them into publishable form. His offer had a profound effect that was entirely symbolic. I never asked for the concrete help he offered, yet his encouraging certainty about the value of my contribution allowed me to begin to write[4].

However, I didn't write in interaction with him or anyone else. Instead, I retreated from the relational arena and entered a space characterized by a (borrowed) illusion of certainty about my work. That contained space temporarily sealed off self-doubt and helped create the feeling of being fully "in my own skin," where I could feel out the edges of my thoughts. In the "being" self-state, I felt identified, even merged, with my supervisor/father.

4  I'm deeply indebted to Larry Epstein for his support.

I embraced myself with his words and on a more unconscious level, evoked the experience of being my father's adored child.

As I wrote my first psychoanalytic paper, then, I bracketed my anxiety about failing in the creative act. When those anxieties resurfaced, I returned to my supervisor to recapture the more insulated "being" self-state, although I seldom engaged in active theoretical dialogue. In this sense, I used a relational experience to support a *retreat* from the very risky relational world.

It's likely that the "being" self-state reflects underlying fears of annihilation, wherein only a complete retreat from the world of real others (and merger with an idealized object) creates a safe arena within which to access creative process. Perhaps this withdrawal is especially necessary for writers whose maternal identification is strong. Historically, cultural forces have located these difficulties within the women's domain; however, I don't believe there's anything intrinsically gendered about them.

In addition to the validation offered by my supervisor (and later by my editor Steve Mitchell and several colleagues), I've used Winnicott as a symbolic psychoanalytic parent whose theoretical concepts supported my thinking. This process wasn't always conscious; I sometimes discovered that I had made use of (and made over) Winnicott's contributions as my own[5].

The illusion of creative certainty represents a retreat from relational challenge. It provides a temporary solution to personal issues that reside in the domain of the legitimacy of subjective process more than interpersonal action. Yet while the "being" illusion excludes the world of threatening objects, there's, perhaps, an implicit (preoedipal) parental identification, even merger, behind this self-state. As I withdrew into myself, I was far from alone; I internalized my supervisor's serene confidence in my creative potential by evoking that (object-related) experience as I wrote.

Over time, validated by some professional successes, I grew more confident. Yet, most paradoxically, as "being" anxieties subsided, I became acutely aware of (and worried about) my place within the professional community. No longer feeling like a child among psychoanalytic adults but instead among peers, I found it more difficult to exclude the threatening Other when I wrote.

---

5 It's notable that a father/mentor was pivotal in facilitating my writing (see Benjamin, 1991).

These were "doing" anxieties; they reflected a worry about the Other—more sibling than parent. At times, these voices were intellectually stimulating; they provoked an internal dialogue that pushed my thinking forward. At other moments, I felt daunted by the wealth of creative analytic writers out there. Aware of the danger of their potential critique, I became stalled, unable to continue articulating my ideas.

To protect myself from these relational anxieties, I sometimes engaged a "doing" fantasy by taking on the relational world in illusory form. In line with Aron's (1995) description, I fantasized my colleagues' admiring (and untextured) responses to my work, the stir it would create. Although this fantasy was more explicitly relational than the "being" illusion, it was no less idealized. It absolutely excluded the likelihood that my papers would be less well received than I hoped or that they would raise questions and criticisms as well as praise.

## The interpenetration of "being" and "doing"

Many writers experience both "being" *and* "doing" anxieties; these two themes represent alternating (rather than alternative) ways of organizing experience. For some (like me), when the basic issue of "being"—that is, of personal legitimacy in the professional world—resolves (what I have to say *is* of value), concerns shift to the "doing" arena (how will my work be received?). For others, these two spheres of concern fluctuate: The writer alternately or simultaneously struggles with "being" and "doing" anxieties. And, of course, each concern can represent a defense against the other. The writer may focus on fears about colleagues' retaliation to sidestep more basic worries about her capacity to think and write, or alternatively, may deny competitive concerns by emphasizing her personal vulnerability. Jane articulated this particularly well:

> Before I start to write I get into this state of anticipatory anxiety about whether the words will flow or not. That anxiety puts me in a negative state where I hugely doubt my creativity. But I also worry about betraying my patients.
>
> Despite the ways that I disguise the material, I worry that they'd be enraged and feel betrayed. Once I get going though, the words flow, and the anxiety disappears. I get into a grandiose, joyous kind of state, thinking this is gonna be great. It's a sort of play, and I'm alone in it. No one is there, it feels incredibly restorative.

When you asked me to tell you about my experience, I had the same reaction—I've already written about this, I have nothing new to say. Then you encouraged me, and I took the step of calling you, and now I feel creative again. It's very close experientially to the sequence that takes place when I try to write.

Jane's retreat to an idealized "being" self-state melds object-related and self-state anxieties. She worries about being inadequate *and* about betraying her patients. Object-related threats thus evoke "being" anxieties and vice versa.

Some writers describe how, when seized by an idea, they must quickly get it down on paper before self-doubt intrudes. Here, the illusion of certainty is accessed only briefly. Still other potential writers find it impossible to begin at all because they can't bracket uncertainty even temporarily. Immobilizing self-doubt, incompatible with the act of creative expression, results in an abandonment of the writing project.

## Idealization and creative rigidity

Despite the potential inherent in creative illusions, they also carry risks. A prolonged retreat to a single-minded illusion of certainty leaves the writer absolutely wedded to her ideas. Vulnerability to critique makes the world of ideas threatening and narrows, even freezes, creative process. Because dialogue with the Other is excluded, the writer remains unprepared for and unable to consider alternative viewpoints.

Unless we can locate our work within the wider world of psychoanalytic ideas, an excessive use of "being" or "doing" illusions, then, limits creative process. Does this issue contribute to the contemporary psychoanalytic phenomenon in which similar processes are described in different language by theoreticians who fail to address or integrate their own perspective within a wider theoretical frame?

It's this tension that I emphasize. When loosely held, creative illusions support the capacity to experience, at alternating moments, self-doubt and a temporary illusion of certainty that are central to a creative and responsive writing process.

## *Postscript*

I wrote this essay more than 30 years ago. Rereading it today, the personal material seems largely historical; my need to retreat to "being" or "doing" self-states has mostly disappeared. That shift reflects, I suspect, time, experience, and positive responses from colleagues. Still, there are moments when I can feel a bit anxious about embarking on a new project. But just a bit; today I can mostly tolerate the relational threats inherent in writing and am able to take on psychoanalytic criticism in the creative moment. Creative space feels genuinely transitional; I enjoy the destruction and reworking of text that are an inevitable part of the writing process[6]. All this has allowed me to read my own work critically without becoming frozen in self-doubt. I can enter the relational arena—literally and symbolically—by turning to other readers for an "objective" (although inevitably subjective) response. What a relief!

Lest you think I'm declaring that I've arrived, let me add that there still are contexts in which I worry about the value of my work and its reception in the professional world. I suspect that these kinds of anxieties will always remain with me. I'm not altogether sorry about that, though. These creative anxieties, while less than pleasant, push me to work longer and harder, to require more of myself than I would in the absence of doubt.

And that, I think, is ultimately a good thing.

---

6 Like most psychoanalytic writers, I've made use of, and implicitly altered, existing theoretical models. Freud (1915), pointing to the creative "invention" involved in theory building, anticipated Bloom's (1973) and Smith's (1997) suggestion that "creative misreading" is intrinsic to the work of the artist and the psychoanalytic writer.

# Afterword

## Against the grain: On challenging assumptions, bridging theories, practicing self-critique, exposing underbellies, and doing the right thing

It's ironic, I think, that so much of my psychoanalytic career focused on the holding theme. Ironic because in the consulting room I rarely work like a Winnicottian. If anything, I tend toward directness; I try hard to find a way to articulate what I'm thinking and why, and I turn to holding reluctantly. So, in a way, I formulated a theory of holding to help me contain *me*, to counterbalance my own preference for unshaded honesty.

The theoretical is, of course, also the personal (Kuchuck, 2013). In part, my attempt to bridge relational and Winnicottian thinking emerged out of a wish (not then conscious) to repair (even undo) my parents' divorce. It also reflected my experience as the mother of three (wonderful but not quite angelic) children. And with some very difficult patients. As both mother and analyst, holding sounded far easier than it turned out to be. And yet, I think it was (and is) essential. I've spent much of my career trying to do all this. Here I offer some thoughts about how and why.

Every chapter in *Psychoanalysis and the Unspoken* questions the assumed and attempts to bridge the apparently incompatible. This has been an intellectual pleasure of mine; I enjoy turning things on their heads, considering both the up- and downside of clinical interventions and addressing the collision between the ideal and the actual. In my view, every theory is vulnerable to exaggerating the value of its position and provoking another pendulum swing. Only self-critique provides an exit from this kind of polarization.

Another theme: Engaging the space between the ideal and the actual. On one hand, our professional ideals support us when the work seems hopeless; they protect us from excessive self-doubt and anxiety. But ideals are also just that; they embed an element of illusion that skips over the collision between how we want/believe we should function and the more imperfect way that we do. Ideals can invite a collusion between patient and analyst; they can result in problematic acting out and/or emotional withdrawal on the analyst's part. In aiming to expose underbellies (especially in Part 2), I consider doing what we feel is the "right thing."

Part 3 addresses a wider range of issues organized around the power—and limits—of illusions and their underbelly. Our own aging, our need to mourn and commemorate across a lifetime, the field's intense infighting, and our capacity to engage in a creative psychoanalytic writing process all explore the up- and downsides of illusion.

In addition to the intellectual sources of these interests, I want to acknowledge and honor my father's indirect contribution to much of this work: He was, in many ways, a bit of an "enfant terrible" who flouted authority, held fast to principles, and refused to conform. He inspired me to do the same.

I end *Psychoanalysis and the Unspoken* by returning to the clinical credo that has guided me across time. It was articulated by my first psychoanalytic mentor, my mother. She was a rule-bound mother, and I was certain she was a rule-bound analyst. But her willingness to step outside her analytic frame to help a patient inspired me as a kid and continues to inspire. Her credo is, I believe, foundational to an ethical psychoanalytic identity; it privileges the "care" element of analytic practice, the value of addressing patient need over theory or clinical rules. To be in the business of helping people above all is my red thread, a credo that has guided and sustained me in the face of its—and my—limitations.

Yes, it's an overly simple credo. It evades complexity—the ways that our beliefs and personal investments color and shape our definition of "help." It implies that our patient's needs are easily identified and unconflicted. It ignores the intersubjective element that can skew our apparently "objective" clinical choice. My mother's choice to get her patient an abortion was certainly not uncomplicated. Still. It's a profoundly ethical ideal that I'm prepared to struggle with and strive for. At 14, I was far too young to appreciate her wisdom or the complexity that lay beneath her simple statement of purpose. I am, alas, no longer too young. And if I can acknowledge and pass on her wisdom to those I train, I'll be more than pleased.

And so, I end with the credo that has guided me across a professional lifetime: Whatever the particulars of your psychoanalytic ideal, find and hold firm to the business you're in—one grounded in an ethic of care. Hold your theory lightly and do your best to remain open to its limitations. Study, question, doubt. Try to retain an ethical stance when expediency would invite you to close your eyes or give in to desire. Above all, enact that ideal by aiming to offer yourself, your wisdom, and your care to your patients ahead of your beliefs, your rules and desires, and your theory, while simultaneously acknowledging the impossibility of this ideal.

# References

Ackerman, S. (2020). Impossible ethics. *JAPA*. 68(4): 561–582, Sept. 2020.

Adler, E., & Bachant, J. L. (1998). Intrapsychic and interactive dimensions of resistance. *Psychoanal. Psych.*, 15: 451–479. doi:10.1037/0736–9735.15.4.451

Ainsworth, M. D. S. (1969). Object relations, dependency, and attachment: A theoretical overview of the infant-mother relationship. *Child Development*, 40(4): 969–1025. doi:10.2307/1127008

Akhtar, S. (2011). *Matters of Life and Death: Psychoanalytic Reflections*. London: Karnac.

Akhtar, S., & Smolar, A. (1998). Visiting the father's grave. *Psychoanal. Quart.*, 67(3): 474–483. https://doi.org/10.1080/00332828.1998.12006052

Alexander, F. (1950). Analysis of the therapeutic factors in psychoanalytic treatment. *Psychoanal. Quart.*, 19: 482–500.

Alpert, J., & Steinberg, A. (Eds.) (2017). Sexual boundary violations. *Psychoanal. Psych.*, 34.

Aron, L. (1991). The patient's experience of the analyst's subjectivity. *Psychoanal. Dial.*, 1: 29–51. doi:10.1080/10481889109538884

Aron, L. (1992). Interpretation as expression of the analyst's subjectivity. *Psychoanal. Dial.*, 2: 475–508.

Aron, L. (1995). The internalized primal scene. *Psychoanal. Dial.*, 5: 195–237.

Aron, L. (1996). *A Meeting of Minds: Mutuality in Psychoanalysis*. Hillsdale, NJ: Analytic Press.

Aron, L. (1999). Clinical choices and the relational matrix. *Psychoanal. Dial.*, 9(1): 1–29.

Aron, L. (2001). *A Meeting of Minds*. NY: Routledge.

Aron, L. (2017). Beyond tolerance in psychoanalytic communities: Reflexive skepticism and critical pluralism. *Psychoanal. Persp.*, 14: 271–282.

Aron, L., Grand, S., & Slochower, J. (2018a). *De-idealizing Relational Theory: A Critique From Within*. London: Routledge.

Aron, L., Grand, S., & Slochower, J. (2018b). *Decentering Relational Theory: A Comparative Critique*. London: Routledge.

Aronson, S. (2009). The (un)designated mourner: When the analyst's patient dies. *Contemp. Psychoanal.*, 45(4): 545–560. https://doi.org/10.1080/00107530.2009.10746028

Ashenburg, K. (2002). *The Mourner's Dance*. Toronto: Macfarlane Walter & Ross.

Bach, S. (1985). *Narcissistic States and the Therapeutic Process*. Northvale, NJ: Aronson.

Balint, M. (1968). *The Basic Fault*. London: Tavistock.

Barwick, N. (2000). Loss, creativity, and leaving home: Investigating adolescent essay anxiety. In: *Clinical Counselling in Schools*, (Ed.) N. Barwick. London: Routledge, pp. 159–174.

Barwick, N. (2003). Mad desire and feverish melancholy: Reflections on the psychodynamics of writing and presenting. *British J. Psychotherapy,* 20: 59–71.

Bass, A. (1996). Holding, holding back, and holding on. Commentary on paper by Joyce Slochower. *Psychoanal. Dial.,* 6: 361–378.

Bass, A. (2001). It takes one to know one; or, whose unconscious is it anyway? *Psychoanal. Dial.,* 11: 683–702.

Bass, A. (2003). "E" enactments in psychoanalysis: Another medium, another message. *Psychoanal. Dial.,* 13: 657–676.

Bassin, D. (1997). Beyond the he and she: Postoedipal transcendence of gender polarities. *JAPA,* 44: 157–190.

Bassin, D. (1998). In Memoriam: "Memorialization" and the working through of mourning. Paper presented at Doris Bernstein Memorial Lecture, Institute for Psychoanalytic Training and Research, and American Psychoanalytic Association Meeting (New York).

Bassin, D. (1999). *Female Sexuality.* Northvale, NJ: Aronson.

Bassin, D. (2003). A not-so-temporary occupation inside Ground Zero. In: J. Greenberg (Ed.), *9/11: Trauma at Home.* Lincoln: University of Nebraska Press.

Bassin, D. (2008). *Leave no Soldier,* documentary. Director and Producer. ShrinkWrap Productions.

Bassin, D., Honey, M., & Kaplan, M. M. (Eds.) (1994). *Representations of Motherhood.* New Haven, CT: Yale Univ. Press.

Baum-Baicker, C. (2018). Defining clinical wisdom. *J. Advancement of Scientific Psychoanal. Empirical Research,* 1(2): 71–83.

Baum-Baicker, C., & Sisti, D. A. (2012). Clinical wisdom in psychoanalysis and psychodynamic psychotherapy: A philosophical and quantitative analysis. *J. Clinical Ethics,* 23: 13–27.

Becker, E. (1973). *The Denial of Death.* NY: Free Press.

Beebe, B., & Lachmann, F. (1994). Representation and internalization in infancy: Three principles of salience. *Psychoanal. Psychol.,* 11(2): 127–165. doi:10.1037/h0 079530

Beebe, B., & Lachmann, F. H. (1998). Co-constructing inner and relational processes. *Psychoanal. Psychol.,* 15: 480–516.

Beebe, B., Lachmann, F., Markese, S., & Bahrick, L. (2012). On the origins of disorganized attachment and internal working models: Paper 1. A dyadic systems approach. *Psychoanal. Dial.,* 22: 253–272.

Benjamin, J. (1986). A desire of one's own: Psychoanalytic feminism and intersubjective space. *Feminist Studies/Critical Studies.* (Ed.) T. de Lauretis. Bloomington: Univ. Indiana Press, pp. 78–101.

Benjamin, J. (1988). *The Bonds of Love: Psychoanalysis, Feminism and the Problem of Domination.* NY: Pantheon.

Benjamin, J. (1991). Father and daughter: Identification with difference—A contribution to gender heterodoxy. *Psychoanal. Dial.,* 1: 277–299.

Benjamin, J. (1995a). *Like Subjects, Love Objects.* New Haven, CT: Yale Univ. Press.

Benjamin, J. (1995b). Sameness and difference: Toward an "overinclusive" model of gender development. *Psychoanal. Inq.,* 15(1): 125–142.

Benjamin, J. (1998). *Shadow of the Other.* London: Routledge.

Benjamin, J. (2009). A relational psychoanalysis perspective on the necessity of acknowledging failure in order to restore the facilitating and containing features of the intersubjective relationship (the shared third). *Int. J. Psycho-Anal.,* 90: 441–450.

Benjamin, J. (2010). Where's the gap and what's the difference? The relational view of intersubjectivity, multiple selves, and enactments. *Contemp. Psychoanal.*, 46: 112–119.

Benjamin, J. (2017). *Beyond Doer and Done to: Recognition Theory, Intersubjectivity, and the Third*. NY: Routledge.

Bergler, E. (1955). Unconscious mechanisms in "writer's block". *Psychoanal. Rev.*, 42: 160–168.

Bergmann, M. S. (1988). On the fate of the intrapsychic image of the psychoanalyst after termination. *Psychoanal. St. Child*, 43: 137–153.

Bergmann, M. S. (1997). Termination: The Achilles heel of psychoanalytic technique. *Psychoanal. Psych.*, 14: 163–174.

Bernstein, J. W. (2000). Making a memorial place: The photography of Shimon Attie. *Psychoanal. Dial.*, 10(3): 347–370. https://doi.org/10.1080/10481881009348551

Bernstein, J. W. (2003). Analytic thefts: Commentary on papers by Joyce Slochower and Sue Grand. *Psychoanal. Dial.*, 13: 501–511. http://dx.doi.org/10.1080/1048188130 9348753

Bion, W. R. (1962). *Learning from Experience*. London: Heinemann.

Bloom, H. (1973). *The Anxiety of Influence*. New York: Oxford Univ. Press.

Bloom, H. (1997). *The Anxiety of Influence*. New Haven: Yale Univ. Press.

Bollas, C. (1987). *The Shadow of the Object*. NY: Col. Univ. Press.

Bollas, C. (1996), Figures and their functions: On the oedipal structure of a psychoanalysis. *Psychoanalytic Quarterly*, 65: 1–20.

Bonovitz, C. (2007). Termination never ends: The inevitable incompleteness of psychoanalysis. *Contemp. Psychoanal.*, 43: 229–246.

Bose, J. (2003). Discussion of Eisold's "The profession of psychoanalysis". *Contemp. Psychoanal.*, 39(4): 583–591.

BPCSG (1998). Non-interpretive mechanisms in psychoanalytic therapy: The "something more" than interpretation. *Int. J. Psycho-Anal.*, 79: 903–921.

Boulanger, G. (2007). *Wounded by Reality: Understanding and Treating Adult-Onset Trauma*. Mahwah, NJ: Analytic Press.

Bromberg, P. M. (1979). Interpersonal psychoanalysis and regression. *Contemp. Psychoanal.*, 15: 647–655.

Bromberg, P. M. (1991). On knowing one's patient inside out: The aesthetics of unconscious communication. *Psychoanal. Dial.*, 1(4): 399–422. https://doi.org/10.1080/1048188910 9538911

Bromberg, P. M. (1993). Shadow and substance: A relational perspective on clinical process. *Psychoanal. Psych.*, 10: 147–168.

Bromberg, P. (1995). Resistance, object-usage, and human relatedness. *Contemp. Psychoanal.*, 31: 173–191.

Bromberg, P. M. (1998). *Standing in the Spaces. Essays on Clinical Process, Trauma and Dissociation*. Hillsdale, NJ: Analytic Press.

Bromberg, P. M. (2006). *Awakening the Dreamer*. Hillsdale, NJ: Analytic Press.

Bromberg, P. M. (2011). *In the Shadow of the Tsunami*. Hillsdale, NJ: Analytic Press.

Buechler, S. (2000). Necessary and unnecessary losses: The analyst's mourning. *Contemp. Psychoanal.*, 36(1): 77–90. https://doi.org/10.1080/00107530.2000.10747046

Celenza, A. (2007). *Sexual Boundary Violations: Therapeutic, Supervisory and Academic Contexts*. Lanham, MD: Aronson.

Celenza, A. (2014). *Erotic Revelations: Clinical Applications and Perverse Scenarios*. London: Routledge.

Celenza, A. (2017). Lessons on or about the couch: What sexual boundary transgressions can teach us about everyday practice. *Psychoanal. Psych.*, 34: 157–162.

Celenza, A. (2021). Shadows that corrupt: Present absences in psychoanalytic process. In: Charles Levin (Ed.), *Boundary Trouble: Psychosexual Violations and Intimacy in Psychoanalysis*, pp. 77–93. NY: Routledge.

Celenza, A. (2022a). Psychoanalysis and #MeToo: Where are we in this movement? *Int. J. of Controversial Discussions*, 2(1): 48–71.

Celenza, A. (2022b). *Transference, Love, Being: Essential Essays from the Field*. London: Routledge.

Celenza, A., & Gabbard, G. O. (2003). Analysts who commit sexual boundary violations: A lost cause? *JAPA*, 51: 617–636.

Chessick, R. D. (1994). On corruption. *J. Amer. Academy Psychoanal.*, 22(3): 377–398.

Chessick, R. D. (2013). Special problems for the elderly psychoanalyst in the psychoanalytic process. *JAPA*, 61, 67–93. doi:10.1177/0003065112474842

Chodorow, N. (1978). *The Reproduction of Mothering*. Berkeley, CA: University of California Press.

Chodorow, N., & Contratto, S. 1982. The fantasy of the perfect mother. In: B. Thorne (Ed.) *Rethinking the Family: Some Feminist Questions*. New York: Longman.

Clough, P. T. (2019). Notes on psychoanalysis and technology: The psychic and the social. *Studies in Gender and Sexuality*, 22: 75–83.

Coltart, N. (1996). *The Baby and the Bathwater*. Madison, CT: Int. Univ. Press.

Cooper, S. (2000). *Objects of Hope*. Hillsdale, NJ: Analytic Press.

Cooper, S. (2014). The things we carry: Finding/creating the object and the analyst's self-reflective participation. *Psychoanal. Dial.*, 24(6): 621–636. https://doi.org/10.1080/104 81885.2014.970963

Cooper, S. (2015). Clinical theory at the border(s): Emerging and unintended crossings in the development of clinical theory. *Int. J. Psycho-Anal.*, 96(2): 273–292.

Corbett, K. (2008). Gender now. *Psychoanal. Dial.*, 18: 838–856.

Corbett, K. (2014). The analyst's private space: Spontaneity, ritual, psychotherapeutic action, and self-care. *Psychoanal. Dial.*, 24(6): 637–647. https://doi.org/10.1080/1048 1885.2014.970964

Craige, H. (2002). Mourning analysis: The post-termination phase. *JAPA*, 50: 507–550.

Craige, H. (2006). Termination, terminable and interminable: Commentary on paper by Jody Messler Davies. *Psychoanal. Dial.*, 16: 585–590.

Crown, N. (2017). Are you sure it was with a patient? What we talk about when we talk about sexual boundary violations. *Psychoanal. Dial.* 27: 71–78.

Csillag, V. (2014). Ordinary sadism in the consulting room. *Psychoanal. Dial.*, 24: 467–482.

Davies, J. M. (1994). Love in the afternoon: A relational reconsideration of desire and dread in the countertransference. *Psychoanal. Dial.*, 4: 153–170.

Davies, J. M. (1998). Multiple perspectives on multiplicity. *Psychoanal. Dial.*, 8: 195–206.

Davies, J. M. (2004). Whose bad objects are we anyway? Repetition and our elusive love affair with evil. *Psychoanal. Dial.*, 14: 711–732.

Davies, J. M. (2005). Transformations of desire and despair: Reflections on the termination process. *Psychoanal. Dial.*, 15: 779–805.

Davies, J. M., & Frawley, M. G. (1994). *Treating Adult Survivor of Childhood Sexual Abuse: A Psychoanalytical Perspective*. NY: Basic Books.

Deri, S. (1976). Transitional Phenomena: Vicissitudes of symbolization and creativity. In: *The Survivor: An Anatomy Life in the Death Camps*, (Ed.) T. Des Press. New York: Oxford Univ. Press.

Deutsch, H. (1973). *The Psychology of Women*. New York: Bantam.

Deutsch, R. A. (2014). *Traumatic Ruptures: Abandonment and Betrayal in the Analytic Relationship*. NY: Routledge.

Dewald, P. A. (1982). Serious illness in the analyst: Transference, countertransference, and reality responses. *JAPA*, 30: 347–363. Doi:10.1177/000306518203000202

Dimen, M. (1991). Deconstructing difference: Gender, splitting, and transitional space. *Psychoanal. Dial.*, 1: 335–353.

Dimen, M. (2011). Lapsus linguae, or a slip of the tongue? A sexual violation in an analytic treatment and its personal and theoretical aftermath. *Contemp. Psychoanal.*, 47: 35–79. Doi:10.1080/00107530.2011.10746441

Dinnerstein, D. (1976). *The Mermaid and the Minotaur*. NY: Harper & Row.

Ehrenberg, D. (1992). *The Intimate Edge*. NY: Norton.

Eigen, M. (1993). *The Electrified Tightrope*. Northvale, NJ: Aronson.

Eisold, K. (1994). The intolerance of diversity in psychoanalytic institutes. *Int. J. Psychoanal.*, 75: 785–780.

Eisold, K. (1998). The splitting of the New York Psychoanalytic Society and the construction of psychoanalytic authority. *Int. J. Psychoanal.*, 79: 871–885.

Engels, R. (2022). The thing with feathers. *Voices: The Art and Science of Psychotherapy*, 58(1): 21–30.

Epstein, L. (1987). The problem of the bad-analyst-feeling. *Modern Psychoanalysis*, 12(1): 35–45.

Epstein, L. (1999). The analyst's "bad-analyst feelings". *Contemp. Psychoanal.*, 35(2): 311–325. Doi:10.1080/ 00107530.1999.10747036

Erikson, E. H. (1950). *Childhood and Society*. NY: Norton.

Erikson, E. H. (1984). Reflections on the last stage—and the first. *Psychoanal. St. Child*, 39: 155–165. Doi:10.1080/00797308.1984.11823424

Erikson, E. H. (1998). *The life cycle completed. Extended version with new chapters on the ninth stage by Joan M. Erikson*. NY: Norton.

Fast, I. (1984). *Gender Identity*. Hillsdale, NJ: Analytic Press.

Firestein, S. K. (1982). Termination of psychoanalysis: Historical, clinical, and pedagogic considerations. *Psychoanal. Inq.*, 2: 473–479.

Fiscalini, J. (1994). Narcissism and coparticipant inquiry: Explorations in contemporary interpersonal psychoanalysis. *Contemp. Psychoanal.*, 30: 747–776.

Fogel, G. I. (1989). The authentic function of psychoanalytic theory: An overview of the contributions of Hans Loewald. *Psychoanaly. Quart.*, 58: 419–451.

Fors, M. (2018). A grammar of power in psychotherapy: Exploring the dynamics of privilege. *American Psychological Association*.

Fors, M. (2019). The implosion of the moral third: Moral omnipotence in the era of horror about Donald Trump. *Studies in Gender and Sexuality*, 20(1), 11–16.

Frankel, J. (2003). Our relationship to analytic ideals: Commentary on papers by Joyce Slochower and Sue Grand. *Psychoanal. Dial.*, 13: 513–520.

Frankiel, R. V. (2007). The long good-bye: Omnipotence, pathological mourning, and the patient who cannot terminate. In: *On Deaths and Endings*, (Eds.) B. Willock, L. C. Bohm, & R. C. Curtis. NY: Routledge, pp. 281–292.

Freud, S. (1896). Further remarks on the neuro-psychoses of defence. *Standard Edition*, III, 157–185. London: Hogarth.

Freud, S. (1914). Remembering, repeating and working-through. *Standard Edition*, 12: 147–156.

Freud, S. (1915). On transience. *Standard Edition*, 14: 305–307.

Freud, S. (1915) The Unconscious. *Standard Edition*, 14: 159–204.

Freud, S. (1916). Some character-types met with in psycho-analytic work. *Standard Edition*, *14*, 309–333.

Freud, S. (1923). The ego and the id. *Standard Edition*, 19, 1–66.

Freud, S. (1926). Inhibitions, symptoms, and anxiety. *Standard Edition*, 20, 87–124.

Freud, S. (1927). The Future of an Illusion. *Standard Edition*, 21: 5–56.

Freud, S. (1929). Letter from Sigmund Freud to Ludwig Binswanger, April 11, 1929. In: *The Letters of Sigmund Freud*. NY: Basic Books, 1960, p. 386.

Freud, S. (1929–1930). *Civilization and Its Discontents*. NY: Norton.

Freud, S. (1937). Analysis terminable and interminable. *Int. J. Psychoanal.*, 18, 373–405.

Freud, S. (1953). The interpretation of dreams. *Standard Edition*, IV. London: Hogarth.

Friedman, G. (1991). Impact of a therapist's life-threatening illness on the therapeutic situation. *Contemp. Psychoanal.*, 27: 405–421. Doi:10.1080/00107530.1991.107 46700

Frommer, M. S. (2005). Living in the liminal spaces of mortality. *Psychoanal. Dial.*, 15(4): 479–498. https://doi.org/10.1080/10481881509348845

Frommer, M. S. (2014). On being an analyst before and after the death of a patient; commentary on a paper by Adam Kaplan. *Psychoanal. Perspect.*, 11(3): 248–256. https://doi.org/ 10.1080/1551806X.2014.938949

Frommer, M. S. (2016). Death is nothing at all: On contemplating non-existence. A relational psychoanalytic engagement of the fear of death. *Psychoanal. Dial.*, 26, 373–390. Doi:10. 1080/10481885.2016.1190599

Gabbard, G. O. (1995a). The early history of boundary violations in psychoanalysis. *JAPA*, 43: 1115–1136. Doi:10.1177/000306519504300408

Gabbard, G. O. (1995b). Countertransference: The emerging common ground. *Int. J. Psychoanal.*, 76: 475–485.

Gabbard, G. O. (2014). Traumatic transmission of sexual boundary violations. Paper presented at Wounds of History Conference, New York, NY.

Gabbard, G. O. (2017). Sexual boundary violations: A thirty-year retrospective. *Psychoanal. Psychol. 34*(2): 151–156. https://doi.org/10.1037/pap0000079

Gabbard, G. O., & Lester, E. (1995). *Boundaries and Boundary Violations in Psychoanalysis*. NY: Basic Books.

Gabbard, G. O., Peltz, M. L., & COPE Study Group on Boundary Violations, Committee on Psychoanalytic Education (2001). Speaking the unspeakable: Institutional reactions to boundary violations by training analysts. *JAPA*, 49: 659–673. http://dx.doi.org/10.11 77/00030651010490020601

Gaines, R. (1997). Detachment and continuity: The two tasks of mourning. *Contemp. Psychoanal.*, 33(4): 549–571. https://doi.org/10.1080/00107530.1997.10747005.

Gay, P. (1968). *Weimar Culture: Outsider as Insider*. NY: Norton.

Gerson, S. (2009). When the third is dead: Memory, mourning, and witnessing in the aftermath of the Holocaust. *Int. J. Psychoanal.*, 90(6): 1341–1357. https://doi.org/10.11 11/j.1745-8315.2009.00214.

Ghent, E. (1992). Paradox and process. *Psychoanal. Dial.*, 2: 135–159.

Goldman, D. (1993) (Ed.). *In One's Bones: The Clinical Genius of Winnicott*. Northvale, NJ: Aronson.

Goldman, D. (2017). *A Beholder's Share: Essays on Winnicott and the Psychoanalytic Imagination*. NY: Routledge.

Goldner, V. (1991). Toward a critical relational theory of gender. *Psychoanal. Dial.*, 1: 249–272.

Goren, E. R. (2017). A call for more talk and less abuse in the consulting room: One psychoanalyst–sex therapist's perspective. *Psychoanal. Psychol.*, 34: 215–220.

Grand, S. (2000). *The Reproduction of Evil*. Hillsdale, NJ: Analytic Press.

Grand, S. (2009). Termination as necessary madness. *Psychoanal. Dial.*, 19: 723–733.

Grand, S. (2010). *The Hero in the Mirror*. NY: Routledge.

Grand, S. (2017b). *The Wounds of History*. NY: Routledge.

Grand, S. (2023). On hatred: Perpetrator fragments and totalitarian objects. *Psychoanal. Dial.*, 33(4): 543–560.

Grand, S., & Salberg, J. (2017). *Transgenerational Trauma and the Other*. NY: Routledge.

Greenberg, J., & Mitchell, S. (1983). *Object Relations in Psychoanalytic Theory*. Boston: Harvard Univ. Press.

Grolnick, S., & Barkin, L. (1978). *Between Reality and Fantasy*. Northvale, NJ: Aronson.

Grossmark, C. (2017). Candidates' responses to sexual boundary violations. *Psychoanal. Dial.*, 7: 79–88.

Grundy, D. (1993). Parricide postponed. *Contemp. Psychoanal.*, 29: 693–710.

Guntrip, H. (1975). My experience of analysis with Fairbairn and Winnicott, *International Review of Psycho-Analysis,* 2: 155.

Hagman, G. (1995a). Death of a selfobject: Toward a self psychology of the mourning process. In: A. Goldberg (Ed.) *The Impact of New Ideas: Progress in Self Psychology,* Volume II (pp. 189–205). Hillsdale, NJ: Analytic Press.

Hagman, G. (1995b). Mourning: A review and reconsideration. *Int. J. Psycho-Anal.*, 76: 909–925. https://pubmed.ncbi.nlm.nih.gov/8926140/

Hagman, G. (1996). The role of the other in mourning. *Psychoanal. Quart.*, 65(2): 327–352. https://doi.org/10.1080/21674086.1996.11927493

Hagman, G. (Ed.) (2016). *New Models of Bereavement Theory and Treatment*. NY: Routledge.

Halbwachs, M. (1992). *On Collective Memory*. Chicago, IL: Univ. Chicago Press.

Hale, N. G., Jr. (1995). *The Rise and Crisis of Psychoanalysis in America: Freud and the Americans, 1917–1985*. New York: Oxford Univ. Press.

Harris, A. (1991). Gender as contradiction. *Psychoanal. Dial.*, 1: 197–224.

Harris, A. (1997). Beyond/outside gender dichotomies. *Psychoanal. Dial.*, 7: 363–366.

Harris, A. (2005). *Gender as Soft Assembly*. Hillsdale, NJ: Analytic Press.

Harris, A. (2009). You must remember this. *Psychoanal. Dial.*, 19: 2–21.

Hesse, E., & Main, M. (2000). Disorganized infant, child, and adult attachment: Collapse in behavioral and attentional strategies. *JAPA*, 48(4): 1097–1128. Doi:10.1177/00030651000480041101

Hirsch, I. (2008). *Coasting in the Countertransference*. NY: Routledge.

Hirsch, I. (2014). *The Interpersonal Tradition: The Origins of Psychoanalytic Subjectivity*. NY: Routledge.

Hoffman, I. Z. (1991). Discussion: Toward a social-constructivist view of the psychoanalytic situation. *Psychoanal. Dial.*, 1: 74–105. Doi:10.1080/10481889109538886

Hoffman, I. Z. (1998). *Ritual and Spontaneity in Psychoanalysis*. Hillsdale, NJ: Analytic Press.

Hoffman, I. Z. (2000). At death's door: Therapists and patients as agents. *Psychoanal. Dial.*, 10: 823–846. Doi:10.1080/10481881009348586

Hoffman, I. Z. (2009). Therapeutic passion in the countertransference. *Psychoanal. Dial.*, 19: 617–637.

Homans, P., & Jonte-Pace, D. (2005). Tracking the emotion in the stone: An essay on psychoanalysis and architecture. *Annual of Psychoanal.*, 33: 261–84.

Honig, R. G., & Barron, J. W. (2013). Restoring institutional integrity in the wake of sexual boundary violations: A case study. *JAPA*, 61: 897–924.

Hornstein, G. A. (2000). *To Redeem One Person is to Redeem the World: A Life of Frieda Fromm-Reichmann*. New York: Free Press.

Ingram, D., & Stine, J. (2016). How senior psychodynamic psychiatrists regard retirement. *Psychodynamic Psychiat.*, 44(2): 211–238. Doi:10.1521/pdps.2016.44.2.211

Issroff, J. (2005). *Donald Winnicott and John Bowlby: Personal and Professional Perspectives*. London: Karen.

Jacobs, T. J. (1983). Dreams and responsibilities: Notes on the making of an institute. *Annual of Psychoanal.*, 11: 29–49.

Jacobs, T. J. (1986). On countertransference enactments. *JAPA*, 34: 289–307.

Jacobs, T. J. (1991). *The Use of the Self: Countertransference and Communication in the Analytic Situation*. NY: Int. Univ. Press.

Janis, I. L. (1972). *Victims of Groupthink: A Psychological Study of Foreign-Policy Decisions and Fiascoes*. Boston: Houghton Mifflin.

Josephs, L. (1995). Countertransference and the analyst's narrative strategies. *Contemp. Psychoanal.*, 31: 345–379.

Kahn, N. E. (2003). Self-disclosure of serious illness: The impact of boundary disruptions for patient and analyst. *Contemp. Psychoanal.*, 39(1): 51–74. Doi:10.1080/00107530.2 003.10747199

Kalb, M. (2015). Ghosts in the consulting room: Reluctant ancestors. *Contemp. Psychoanal.*, 51(1): 74–106. Doi:10.1080/00107530.2015.985905

Kalb, M. (2021). On ghosts: An aspect of the universal infantile and its theoretical-clinical perils and promises. Paper presented at 52nd Congress of International Psychoanalytical Association, online, July 23.

Kalb, M. (in press). Hans W. Loewald: Quiet revolutionary, creative synthesizer, inspiration for 21st century psychoanalysis. An introduction to the Hans W. Loewald Center. In: Balsam, R., Brett, E., & Levenson L. (Eds.) *The Emerging Tradition of Hans Loewald*. London: Routledge.

Kantrowitz, J. l. (2015). *Myths of Termination: What Patients Can Teach Psychoanalysts about Endings*. NY: Routledge.

Kernberg, O. F. (1974). Further contributions to the treatment of narcissistic personalities. *Int. J. Psycho-Anal.*, 55: 215–240.

Kernberg, O. F. (1986). Institutional problems of psychoanalytic education. *J. Amer. Psychoanal. Assn.*, 34: 799–834.

Kernberg, O. F. (1996). Thirty methods to destroy the creativity of psychoanalytic candidates. *Int. J. Psycho-Anal.*, 77: 1031–1040.

Kernberg, O. F. (2000). A concerned critique of psychoanalytic education. *Int. J. Psycho-Anal.*, 81: 97–120.

Kirsner, D. (1990). Mystics and professionals in the culture of American psychoanalysis. *Free Associations*, 1(20): 85–103.

Klass, D. (1988). *Parental Grief: Solace & Resolution*. NY: Springer.

Klein, M. (1948). A contribution to the theory of anxiety and guilt. *Int. J. Psycho-Anal.*, 29: 114–123.

Klein, M. (1975). *Envy and Gratitude and Other Works* 1946–1963. Int. Psychoanalytical Library (Vol. 104, pp. 1–346). London: Hogarth.

Kohut, H. (1971). *The Analysis of the Self*. NY: Int. Univ. Press.

Kohut, H. (1977). *The Restoration of the Self*. NY: Int. Univ. Press.

Kohut, H. (1984). *How Does Analysis Cure*. Chicago, IL: University of Chicago Press.

Kohut, T. A. (2020). History flows through us: Psychoanalysis, historical trauma, and the shaping of experience. *Psychoanalysis, Self, and Context*, 15: 20–24.

Kraemer, S. (1996). "Betwixt the dark and the daylight" of maternal subjectivity: Meditations on the threshold. *Psychoanal. Dial.*, 6: 765–791.

Kraemer, D. (2000). *Meanings of Death in Rabbinic Judaism*. London: Routledge.

Kubie, L. S. (1968). Unsolved problems in the resolution of the transference. *Psychoanal. Quart.*, 37: 331–352.

Kuchuck, S. (2013). *Clinical Implications of the Psychoanalyst's Life Experience: When the Personal Becomes Professional*. London: Karnac.

Kumin, I. (1985–1986). Erotic horror: Desire and resistance in the psychoanalytic situation. *Int. J. Psychoanal. Psychotherapy*, 11: 3–25.

Kuriloff, E. (2010). The holocaust and psychoanalytic theory and praxis. *Contemp. Psychoanal.*, 46(3): 395–422.

Lamm, M. (1988). *The Jewish Way in Death and Mourning*. New York: Jonathan David.

Laub, D. (1992). Bearing witness: Or the vicissitudes of listening. In: Felman, S., Laub, D., (Eds.) *Testimony: Crises of Witnessing in Literature, Psychoanalysis, and History*, (pp. 57–74). NY: Routledge.

Laub, D., & Auerhahn, N. C. (1993). Knowing and not knowing massive psychic trauma. Forms of traumatic memory. *Int. J. Psycho-Anal.*, 74: 287–302.

Laub, D., & Podell, D. (1995). Art and trauma. *Int. J. Psycho-Anal.*, 76: 995–1005.

Layton, L. (1998), *Who's that Girl? Who's that Boy? Clinical Practice Meets Post-Modern Gender Theory*. Northvale, NJ: Aronson.

Layton, L. (2010). Maternal resistance. In: (Ed.) J. Salberg, *Good Enough Endings*. NY: Routledge, pp. 191–210.

Lazarre, J. (1976). *The Mother Knot*. New York: Dell.

Levine, H. B., & Yanof, J. A. (2004). Boundaries and postanalytic contacts in institutes. *JAPA*, 52: 873–901.

Levi-Strauss, C. (1985). *A View from Afar*. NY: Basic Books.

Little, M. (1990). *Psychotic Anxieties and Containment*. Northvale, NJ: Aronson.

Lobban, G. (2007). Reclaiming the relationship with the lost parent following parental death during adolescence. In: B. Willock, L. C. Bohm, & R. C. Curtis (Eds.), *On Deaths and Endings*. London: Routledge, pp. 131–145.

Loewald, H. W. (1960). On the therapeutic action of psycho-analysis. *Int. J. Psycho-Anal.*, 41: 16–33.

Loewald, H. (1962). Internalization, separation, mourning and the superego. *Psychoanal. Quart.*, 31: 483–504.

Loewald, H. (1972). The experience of time. *Psychoanal. St. Child*, 27: 401–410. doi:10.10 80/00797308.1972.11822722

Loewald, H. (1976). Perspectives on memory. In: *Papers on Psychoanalysis*. New Haven, CT: Yale Univ. Press, pp. 148–173.

Loewald, H. (1979). The waning of the Oedipus complex. *JAPA*, 27: 751–776.

Loewald, H. W. (1988). Termination analyzable and unanalyzable. *Psychoanal. St. Child*, 43: 155–166.

Lyons, L. (2014). Growing up in the old left: An intergenerational tale of silence and terror. *Studies in Gender and Sexuality*, 15: 182–198. doi:10.1080/15240657.2014.939019

Mahler, M. (1968). On human symbiosis and the vicissitudes of individuation. *JAPA*, 15: 740–763.

Mandelbaum, D. G. (1959). Social uses of funeral rites. In: Feifel, H. (Ed.) *The Meaning of Death*. NY: McGraw-Hill, pp. 189–217.

Margolis, M. (1997). Analyst-patient sexual involvement: Clinical experiences and institutional responses. *Psychoanal. Inq.*, 17: 349–370. doi:10.1080/07351699709534131

McKay, R. K. (2019). Where objects were subjects now may be: The work of Jessica Benjamin and reimagining maternal subjectivity in transitional space. *Psychoanal. Inq.*, 39: 163–173.

McWilliams, N. (2004). *Psychoanalytic Psychotherapy: A Practitioner's Guide*. New York, London: Guilford.

McWilliams, N. (2011). *Psychoanalytic Diagnosis*. NY: Guilford.

McWilliams, N. (2017). Psychoanalytic reflections on limitation: Aging, dying, generativity and renewal. *Psychoanal. Psychol.*, 34(1): 50–57. doi:10.1037/pap0000107

Mitchell, S. (1984). Object relations theories and the developmental tilt. *Contemp. Psychoanal.*, 20: 473–499.

Mitchell, S. (1988). *Relational Concepts in Psychoanalysis*. Cambridge, MA: Harvard Univ. Press.

Mitchell, S. (1991). Wishes, needs and interpersonal negotiations. *Psychoanal. Inq.*, 11: 147–170.

Mitchell, S. (1993). *Hope and Dread in Psychoanalysis*. NY: Basic Books.

Mitchell, S. (1997). *Influence and Autonomy in Psychoanalysis*. Hillsdale, NJ: Analytic Press.

Mitchell, S. (2000). *Relationality*. Hillsdale, NJ: Analytic Press.

Modell, A. H. (1975). A narcissistic defense against affects and the illusion of self sufficiency. *Int. J. Psycho-Anal.*, 56: 275–282.

Modell, A. H. (1976). The holding environment and the therapeutic action of psychoanalysis. *JAPA*, 24: 285–307.

Modell, A. H. (1990). *Other Times, Other Realities: Toward a Theory of Psychoanalytic Treatment*. Cambridge, MA: Harvard Univ. Press.

Modell, A. (1990). Transference and levels of reality. In: A. Modell, *Other Times, Other Realities* (pp. 44–59). Cambridge, MA: Harvard Univ. Press.

Morrison, A. (1989). *Shame: The Underside of Narcissism*. Hillsdale, NJ: Analytic Press.

Morrison, A. (1997). Ten years of doing psychotherapy while living with a life threatening illness: Self-disclosure and other ramifications. *Psychoanal. Dial.*, 7: 225–241. doi:10.1080/10481889709539178

Nass, M. L. (2015). The omnipotence of the psychoanalyst: Thoughts on the need to consider retirement. *JAPA*, 63: 1013–1023. doi:10.1177/0003065115609445

Nora, P. (Ed.). (1989). Between Memory and History: Les Lieux de Mémoire (1984). *Representations*, 26: 7–25.

Nora, P., (Ed.) (1984–1992). *Les Lieux de Mémoire*. 7 vols. Paris: Éditions Gallimard.

Ogden, T. H. (1986). *The Matrix of the Mind*. NY: Jason Aronson.

Ogden, T. H. (1989). *The Primitive Edge of Experience*. NY: Jason Aronson.

Ogden, T. H. (1994). The analytic third: Working with intersubjective clinical facts. *Int. J. Psycho-Anal.*, 75: 3–19.

Ogden, T. H. (1994). *Subjects of Analysis*. NY: Routledge.

Ogden, T. H. (1997). Reverie and metaphor: Some thoughts on how I work as a psychoanalyst. *Int. J. Psycho-Anal.*, 78: 719–732.

Orange, D. M. (2008). Whose shame is it anyway? *Contemp. Psychoanal.*, 44: 83–100.

Orfanos, S. D. (1997). Mikis Theodorakis: Music, culture, and the creative process. *J. Modern Hellenism.* 14: 17–37.

Orfanos, S. D. (1999). The creative boldness of Mikis Theodorakis. *J. Modern Hellenism,* 16: 27–39.

Ornstein, A. (2008). Artistic creativity and the healing process. *Psychoanal. Inq.,* 26: 386–406.

Pedder, J. R. (1988). Termination reconsidered. *Int. J. Psycho-Anal.,* 69: 495–505.

Pepper, R. S. (2014). *Emotional Incest in Group Psychotherapy.* London: Rowman & Littlefield.

Pfeffer, A. Z. (1963). The meaning of the analyst after analysis: A contribution to the theory of therapeutic results. *JAPA,* 11: 229–244.

Pizer, B. (1997). When the analyst is ill: Dimensions of self-disclosure. *Psychoanal. Quart.,* 66, 450–469.

Pizer, B. (2000). The therapist's routine consultations: A necessary window in the treatment. *Psychoanal. Dial.,* 10: 197–207. http://dx.doi.org/10.1081/10481881009348531

Pizer, S. A. (1992). The negotiation of paradox in the analytic process. *Psychoanal. Dial.,* 2: 215–240.

Pizer, S. A. (1998). *Building Bridges.* Hillsdale, NJ: Analytic Press.

Pizer, S. A. (2009). Inside out: The state of the analyst and the state of the patient. *Psychoanal. Dial.,* 19(1): 49–62. Doi:10.1080/10481880802634693

Powell, D. R. (2018). Race, African Americans, and psychoanalysis: Collective silence in the therapeutic situation. *JAPA,* 66(6).

Prince, R. (2009). Psychoanalysis traumatized: The legacy of the holocaust. *Amer. J. Psychoanal.,* 69(3): 179–194

Rangell, L. (1983). Defense and resistance in psychoanalysis and life. *JAPA,* 31: 147–174.

Reich, A. (1958). A special variation of technique. *Int. J. Psycho-Anal.,* 39: 230–234.

Reich, W. (1975). *Character Analysis.* New York: Farrar.

Reiner, A. & Bail. B. W. (1997). Infancy and the essential nature of work. In: *Work and its Inhibitions,* (Ed.) C. W. Socarides, & S. Kramer. Madison, CT: International Universities Press, pp. 61–78.

Renik, O. (1991). One kind of negative therapeutic reaction. *JAPA,* 39: 87–105.

Renik, O. (1995). The role of an analyst's expectations in clinical technique: Reflections on the concept of resistance. *JAPA,* 43: 83–94. doi:10.1177/000306519504300108

Renik, O. (1996). The analyst's self-discovery. *Psychoanal. Inq.,* 16: 390–400.

Renik, O. (1999). Getting real in psychoanalysis. *J. Anal. Psych.,* 44: 167–187.

Rosenblum, R. (2009). Postponing trauma. *Int. J. Psycho-Anal.,* 90(6): 1319–1340.

Rubin, S. (1985). The resolution of bereavement: A clinical focus on the relationship to the deceased. *Psychotherapy: Theory, Research, Training and Practice,* 22(2): 231–35.

Salberg, J. (2009). Leaning into termination. *Psychoanal. Dial.,* 19: 704–722.

Salberg, J. (Ed.). (2010). *Good Enough Endings.* NY: Routledge.

Salberg, J. (Ed.) (2022). *Psychoanalytic Credos: Personal and Professional Journeys of Psychoanalysts.* NY: Routledge, pp. 142–151.

Sandler, J. (1960). The background of safety. *Int. J. Psycho-Anal.,* 41: 352–356.

Sandler, J. (1976). Countertransference and role-responsiveness. *Int. J. Psycho-Anal.,* 3: 43–47.

Sandler, A. M., & Godley, W. (2004). Institutional responses to boundary violations: The case of Masud Khan. *International Journal of Psychoanalysis, 85*: 27–43. http://dx.doi.org/10.1516/LP8G-5A70-9FFR-U62Q

Sandler, J. (1983). Reflections on some relations between psychoanalytic concepts and psychoanalytic practice. *Int. J. Psychoanal.*, 64: 35–45.

Schachter, J. (1992). Concepts of termination and post-termination patient-analyst contact. *Int. J. Psycho-Anal.*, 73: 137–154.

Schachter, J. (2005). Postanalytic contacts in institutes. *JAPA*, 53: 260–264.

Schore, A. N. (2003a). *Affect Dysregulation and Disorders of the Self.* NY: Norton.

Schore, A. N. (2003b). *Affect Regulation and the Repair of the Self.* NY: Norton.

Schore, A. N. (2011). The right brain implicit self lies at the core of psychoanalysis. *Psychoanal. Dial.*, 21: 75–100.

Seligman, S. (2003). The developmental perspective in relational psychoanalysis. *Contemp. Psychoanal.*, 39: 477–508.

Seligman, S. (2012). The baby out of the bathwater: Microseconds, psychic structure, and psychotherapy. *Psychoanal. Dial.*, 22: 499–509.

Seligman, S. & Shanok, R. S. (1996). Erikson, our contemporary: His anticipation of an intersubjective perspective. *Psychoanal. Contemp. Thought*, 19: 339–365.

Shabad, P. (2001). *Echoes of Mourning in Psychotherapy.* Northvale, NJ: Aronson.

Shepard, O. (Ed.) (1961). *The Heart of Thoreaus's Journals.* NY: Dover Publications.

Siggins, L. D. (1966). Mourning: A critical survey of the literature. *Int. J. Psycho-Anal.*, 47(1): 14–25. https://pep-web.org/browse/ijp/volumes/47?preview=IJP.047.0014A

Silverman, P. R., Nickman, S., & Worden, J. W. (1992). Detachment revisited: The child's reconstruction of a dead parent. *Amer. J. Orthopsychiatry*, 62(4): 494–503.

Slavin, M. O. & Kriegman, D. (1998). Why the analyst needs to change: Toward a theory of conflict, negotiation, and mutual influence in the therapeutic process. Psychoanal. Dial., 8: 247–284.

Slochower, J. (1991). Variations in the analytic holding environment. *Int. J. Psycho-Anal.*, 72, 709–718.

Slochower, J. (1992). A hateful borderline patient and the holding environment. *Contemp. Psychoanal.*, 28(1): 72–88. https://doi.org/10.1080/00107530.1992.10746738

Slochower, J. (1993). Mourning and the holding function of shiva. *Contemp. Psychoanal.*, 30(1): 135–151. https://doi.org/10.1080/00107530.1994.10746846

Slochower, J. (1994). The evolution of object usage and the holding environment. *Contemp. Psychoanal.*, 30(1): 135–151.

Slochower, J. (1995). The therapeutic function of shiva. In: J. Reimer (Ed.) *Wrestling with the Angel.* NY: Schocken Books.

Slochower, J. (1996a). Holding and the evolving maternal metaphor. *Psychoanal. Rev.*, 83(2): 195–218.

Slochower, J. (1996b). The holding environment and the fate of the analyst's subjectivity. *Psychoanal. Dial.*, 6(3): 323–353. https://doi.org/10.1080/10481889609539123

Slochower, J. (1996c, 2014b, 2014d). *Holding and Psychoanalysis: A Relational Perspective.* NY: Routledge.

Slochower, J. (1998a). Clinical controversies: Ending an analytic relationship. *Psychologist-Psychoanalyst*, 24–25.

Slochower, J. (1998b). Illusion and uncertainty in psychoanalytic writing. *Int. J. Psycho-Anal.*, 79: 333–347.

Slochower, J. (1999). Interior experience in analytic process. *Psychoanal. Dial.*, 9(6): 789–809. https://doi.org/10.1080/10481889909539362

Slochower, J. (2004). But what do *you* want? The location of emotional experience. *Contemp. Psychoanal.*, 40(4): 577–602. https://doi.org/10.1080/00107530.2004.10747245

Slochower, J. (2006c). Holding: something old and something new. In Aron, L. & Harris, A. (Eds.) *Relational Psychoanalysis: Innovation and Expansion*, II: 29–50.

Slochower, J. (2010). Jewish ritual through a psychoanalytic lens. In: L. Aron & L. Henik (Eds.), *Answering a Question with a Question* (pp. 105–128). Brighton, MA: Academic Studies Press.

Slochower, J. (2011a). Out of the analytic shadow: On the dynamics of commemorative ritual. *Psychoanal. Dial.*, 21(6): 676–690. https://doi.org/10.1080/10481885.2011. 629565

Slochower, J. (2011b). Analytic idealizations and the disavowed: Winnicott, his patients, and us. *Psychoanal. Dial.*, 21, 3–21. doi:10.1080/10481885.2011.545317

Slochower, J. (2013). Using Winnicott today: A relational perspective. *Revue Roumaine de Psychanalyse*. 2: 13–41.

Slochower, J. (2013c). Analytic enclaves and analytic outcome: A clinical mystery. *Psychoanal. Dial.*, 23(2): 243–258. https://doi.org/10.1080/10481885.2013.772485

Slochower, J. (2014b). Psychoanalytic mommies and psychoanalytic babies: A long view. *Contemp. Psychoanal.*, 49: 606–628.

Slochower, J. (2014a). Analytic sadism and analytic restraint. *Psychoanal. Dial.*, 24: 483–487.

Slochower, J. (2014c). *Psychoanalytic Collisions*. Hillsdale, NJ: Analytic Press. (Original work published 2006.)

Slochower, J. (2014d). Idéalizations analytiques et le disavoué: Winnicott, ses patients, et nous. *Revue Francaise De Psychanalyse*, 78(4): 1136–1149. https://doi.org/10.3917/ rfp.784.1136

Slochower, J. (2015a). Across a lifetime: On the dynamics of commemorative ritual. In: L. Aron & L. Henik (Eds.), *Answering a Question with a Question* (Vol. II, pp. 273–297). Academic Studies Press.

Slochower, J. (2015b). *Collisioni Psicoanalitiche*. Milano, Ferrari Sinibaldi.

Slochower, J. (2017). Going too far: Relational heroines and relational excess. *Psychoanal. Dial.*, 27, 282–299.

Slochower, J. (2017a). Analisti genitori e pazienti e bambini? Un'indagine retrospettiva. *Ricerca Psicoanalitica*, 1: 9–32.

Slochower, J. (2017b). Don't tell anyone. *Psychoanal. Psychol.*, 34: 195–200.

Slochower, J. (2017c). Introduction to panel: Ghosts that haunt: Sexual boundary violations in our communities. *Psychoanal, Dial.*, 27: 61–66.

Slochower, J. (2018a). Mamás psicoanalíticas y bebés psicoanalíticos: Una visión ampliada. *Clínica E Investigación Relacional*, 12(3): 444–464. https://doi.org/10.21110/19882939 .2018.120303

Slochower, J. (2019). Getting better all the time? *Psychoanal. Dial.*, 29: 548–559.

Slochower, J. (2020). Resist this. *Psychoanal. Dial.*, 30, 64–72.

Slochower, J. (2020). Binaries, dialectics, and their value. In: *When Minds Meet: The Work of Lewis Aron*, G. Atlas (Ed). NY: Routledge.

Slochower, J. (2022a). Against the grain: On challenging assumptions, bridging theories, practicing self-critique, exposing underbellies, and doing the right thing. In Salberg, J. (Ed.)

(2022). *Psychoanalytic Credos: Personal and Professional Journeys of Psychoanalysts.* NY: Routledge, pp. 142–151.

Slochower, J. (2022b). A few regrets. *Psychoanal. Dial.,* 31(2): 166–180.

Slochower, J. (2022b, c). The absent witness: Mourning, virtually. *Psychoanal. Perspect.,* 19(3): 253–268.

Smith, H. F. (1997). Creative misreading: Why we talk past each other. *JAPA,* 45: 335–357.

Solomon, M. (1995). *Mozart.* NY: Harper Collins.

Sorenson, R. L. (2000). Psychoanalytic institutes as religious denominations: Fundamentalism, progency, and ongoing reformation. *Psychoanal. Dial.,* 10: 847–874.

Spezzano, C. (1998). Listening and interpreting—how relational analysts kill time between disclosures and enactments: Commentary on papers by Bromberg and by Greenberg. *Psychoanal. Dial.,* 8: 237–246.

Stein, R. (1997). The shame experiences of the analyst. *Progress in Self Psychology,* 13: 109–123.

Stein, R. (1999). Discussion of Joyce Slochower's Interior experience paper. *Psychoanal. Dial.,* 9: 811–823.

Stein, R. (2008). The Otherness of Sexuality: Excess. *JAPA,* 56(1): 43–71.

Stern, D. (1985). *The Interpersonal World of the Infant: A View from Psychoanalysis and Developmental Psychology.* NY: Basic Books.

Stern, D. B. (1992). Commentary on constructivism in clinical psychoanalysis. *Psychoanal. Dial.,* 2(3): 331–364. https://doi.org/10.1080/10481889209538937

Stern, D. B. (1997). *Unformulated Experience: From Dissociation to Imagination in Psychoanalysis.* Hillsdale, NJ: Analytic Press.

Stern, D. B. (2009). *Partners in Thought.* NY: Routledge.

Stern, D. B. (2015). Relational Freedom: Emergent Properties of the Interpersonal Field. NY: Routledge.

Stern, D. N. (2004). *The Present Moment in Psychotherapy and Everyday Life.* NY: Norton.

Stern, S. (1994). Needed relationships and repeated relationships: An integrated relational perspective. *Psychoanal. Dial.,* 4: 317–346.

Stern, S. (2020). Analytic adoption of the psychically homeless. *Psychoanalysis, Self, and Context,* 16(1): 24–42.

Sternberg, R. J. (2003). *Wisdom, Intelligence, and Creativity Synthesized.* New York: Cambridge University Press.

Stolorow, R. D. (1997). Dynamic, dyadic, intersubjective systems: An evolving paradigm for psychoanalysis. *Psychoanal. Psychol.,* 14: 337–346. doi:10.1037/h0079729

Stolorow, R. D., & Atwood, G. E., (1992). *Contexts of Being.* Hillsdale, NJ: Analytic Press.

Suleiman, S. R. (1985), Writing and motherhood. In: *The (M)other Tongue,* (Ed.) S. N. Garner, C. Kahane, & M. Sprengnether. Ithaca, NY: Cornell University Press.

Suler, J. (2005). The Online Disinhibition Effect. *International Journal of Applied Psychoanalytic Studies,* 2: 184–188

Sullivan, H. S. (1954). *The Psychiatric Interview.* NY: Norton.

Tessman, L. H. (2003). *The Analyst's Analyst Within.* Hillsdale, NJ: Analytic Press.

Trub, L. (2021). Playing and digital reality: Treating kids and adolescents in a pandemic. *Psychoanal. Perspect.,* 18(2): 208–225. https://doi.org/10.1080/1551806X.2021.1896308

Trub, L. (2023). Imagination foreclosed: Searching for each other in the digital age. *Psychoanal. Perspect.,* 20:2, 146–169. doi:10.1080/1551806X.2023.2188026

Trub, L., & Magaldi, D. (2017). Left to our own devices. *Psychoanal. Perspect.*, 14(2): 219–236. https://doi.org/10.1080/1551806X.2017.1304118

Viorst, J. (1986). *Necessary Losses*. New York: Simon & Schuster.

Volkan, V. (1981). *Linking Objects and Linking Phenomena*. NY: Int. Univ. Press.

Volkan, V. (2007). Individuals and societies as "perennial mourners" their linking objects and public memorials. In B. Willock, L. Bohm, & R. Curtis (Eds.) *On Deaths and Endings* (pp. 42–59). NY: Routledge.

Wallerstein, R. (1986). The termination of the training analysis: The process, the expectations, the achievement. The institute's view. In: *The Termination of the Training Analysis: Process: Expectations, Achievements.*, (Ed.) A. Cooper. London: International Psychoanalytical Association, pp. 542–567.

Wallerstein, R. S. (1990). Psychoanalysis: The common ground. *Int. J. Psycho-Anal.*, 71(3): 20.

Warshaw, S. C. (1992). Mutative factors in child psychoanalysis: A comparison of diverse relational perspectives. In: Skolnick, N. & Warshaw, S. C. (Eds.) *Relational Perspectives in Psychoanalysis*. Hillsdale. NJ: Analytic Press.

Weinshel, E., & Renik, O. (1991). The past ten years: Psychoanalysis in the United States, 1980–1990. *Psychoanal. Inq.*, 11: 13–29.

Willock, B. (2007). *Comparative-Integrative Psychoanalysis: A Relational Perspective for the Discipline's Second Century/Edition 1*. New York: Taylor & Francis.

Wilson, M. (2003). The analyst's desire and the problem of narcissistic resistances. *JAPA*, 51: 71–99.

Wilson, M. (2020). And let me go on: Desire and the ending of analysis. In Wilson, J. (2021). *The Analyst's Desire: The Ethical Foundation of Clinical Practice*. NY: Bloomsbury Academic Press, pp. 195–210.

Winnicott, D. W. W. (1947). Hate in the countertransference. In: *Through Pediatrics to Psychoanalysis* (1958). NY: Basic Books.

Winnicott, D. W. W. (1949). The use of an object and relating through identifications. *Playing and Reality*. NY: Basic Books, 86–94.

Winnicott, D. W. W. (1951). Transitional objects and transitional phenomenon. In: *Through Pediatrics to Psychoanalysis* (pp. 229–242). NY: Basic Books.

Winnicott, D. W. W. (1955). Metapsychological and clinical aspects of regression within the psycho-analytical set-up. *Int. J. Psycho-Anal.*, 36: 16–26.

Winnicott, D. W. W. (1958). The capacity to be alone. In: *The Maturational Processes and the Facilitating Environment* (pp. 29–36). NY: Int. Univ. Press, 1965.

Winnicott, D. W. W. (1960a). Ego distortions in terms of true and false self. In: *The Maturational Processes and the Facilitating Environment* London: Hogarth, pp. 147–152.

Winnicott, D. W. W. (1960b). The theory of the parent-infant relationship. In: *The Maturational Processes and the Facilitating Environment*. NY: Int. Univ. Press, 1965, pp. 37–55.

Winnicott, D. W. W. (1962). The aims of psychoanalytical treatment. In *The Maturational Processes and the Facilitating Environment*. NY: Routledge, 2018, pp. 166–170.

Winnicott, D. W. W. (1963a). Dependence in infant care, in child-care, and in the psychoanalytic setting. *Int. J. Psycho-Anal.*, 44: 339–344.

Winnicott, D. W. W. (1963b). From dependence towards independence in the development of the individual. In *Maturational processes and the facilitating environment* (pp. 83–92). London: Hogarth.

Winnicott, D. W. W. (1964). *The Child, the Family, and the Outside World*. London: Perseus.

Winnicott, D. W. W. (1965). *The Maturational Processes and the Facilitating Environment.* London: Hogarth.

Winnicott, D. W. W. (1970). *Home is Where We Start from*. NY: Norton.

Winnicott, D. W. W. (1971). *Playing and Reality*. NY: Basic Books.

Winnicott, D. W. W. (1975). Primary maternal preoccupation. In *Through Pediatrics to Psychoanalysis*. NY: Basic Books.

Winnicott, D. W. W. (1986). *Holding and interpretation: Fragments of an analysis.* London: Karnac.

Witenberg, E. (1976). Termination is no end. *Contemp. Psychoanal.*, 12: 335–338.

Wolstein, B. (1959). *Counter-Transference*. NY: Grune & Stratton.

Yanof, J. A., & Levine, H. B. (2005). Judith A. Yanof and Howard B Levine respond. *JAPA*, 53: 264–265.

Yerushalmi, Y. H. (1982). Zakhor: Jewish History and Jewish Memory. Washington, DC: Univ. of Washington Press.

Young-Bruehl, E., & Schwartz, M. M. (2012). Why psychoanalysis has no history. *Amer. Imago*, 69(1): 139–159.

Zerubavel, Y. (1995). *Recovered Roots: Collective Memory and the Making of Israeli National Tradition*. Chicago, IL: Univ. Chicago Press.

# Author bios

**Nancy McWilliams** is Visiting Professor Emerita at Rutgers Graduate School of Applied & Professional Psychology and has a private practice in Lambertville, NJ. She is author of four textbooks (on psychoanalytic diagnosis, case formulation, therapy, and supervision) and is co-editor of both editions of the *Psychodynamic Diagnostic Manual*. A former president of the Society for Psychoanalysis and Psychoanalytic Psychotherapy of the American Psychological Association, she is a member of the Austen Riggs Center Board of Trustees. Her books are available in 20 languages, and she has taught in 30 countries.

**Dodi Goldman**, Ph.D. is a Training and Supervising Analyst and Faculty at the William Alanson White Institute. He authored, *In Search of the Real: The Origins and Originality of D.W. Winnicott,* edited and wrote an introduction to *In One's Bones: The Clinical Genius of D.W. Winnicott,* and is the former book review editor of the journal *Contemporary Psychoanalysis.* His book, *A Beholder's Share: Essays on Winnicott and the Psychoanalytic Imagination,* won the 2017 Gradiva Award for Best Psychoanalytic Book. A forthcoming book, *A Shimmering Landscape: The Imaginative and Actual in Psychic Life* will be published by Routledge in 2025. Dodi maintains a private practice and study groups in Manhattan and Great Neck, NY.

**Andrea Celenza**, Ph.D. is a Training and Supervising Analyst at the Boston Psychoanalytic Society and Institute and Assistant Clinical Professor at Harvard Medical School. She is also Adjunct Faculty at the NYU Post-Doctoral Program in Psychoanalysis and The Florida Psychoanalytic Center. She has written numerous papers on love, sexuality, and psychoanalysis. She has two online courses and is the recipient of several awards. Her writings have been translated into Italian, Spanish, Korean, Russian, and Farsi. Her third book, entitled, *Transference, Love, and Being: Essential Essays from the Field,* was published in 2022 by Routledge. Dr. Celenza is in private practice in Lexington, Massachusetts, USA.

**Irwin Kula** is a seventh generation rabbi, President Emeritus of Clal— The National Jewish Center for Learning and Leadership and author of the award-winning book *Yearnings: Embracing the Sacred Messiness of Life.* He works with organizations, foundations, and businesses around the world at the intersection of religion, innovation, and the sciences of human flourishing. A commentator in both new and traditional media, he is cofounder with Craig Hatkoff and the late Professor Clay Christensen of the Disruptor Foundation whose mission is to advance disruptive innovation theory and its application in societal critical domains. Irwin lives in NYC. His most important teachers and greatest joys are his wife of 41 years, his two daughters and sons-in-law, and his two grandchildren, the elder of whom regularly says, "I can do it by my own self."

# Index

abandonment: of concepts 28, 142, 179; early experiences of 55, 59; of ethics 79, 90; fear of 54; of ideal 84, 177; of patient feelings of 36, 61, 135; of patients 75, 77; of victims 86; of writing 192, 199
abortion 177, 202
absence 7, 46, 57, 61, 161; of analytic other 114; of capacity 10; connections 133; of death 151, 153; element 164; emotional 192; of emotional demands 75; ghostly 110; of grief 149; intolerable 163; mother 24; object 112; and presence 156, 159, 165; of relationships 107; of responsive other 16; of separateness 115; surrender to 125; of visual stimulation 77
abstinent 41, 43, 178; see also classical
activism 163, 167
adult 9, 23, 28–29, 62; adulthood 24, 68, 155; experiences 14, 59; function 41; need for repair 45; shadow of baby 22; states 21, 57–58; vulnerability 131
affect regulation: developing 61, 116, 141; difficulties involving 18, 34, 59; down-regulation 11; and holding 53, 60; self 16, 22, 62, 64, 83; by therapist 17
agency 36, 38, 60, 107, 131; and aging 132; development of 62, 107, 116, 163; emotional 59; ethical 88, 90; undermine 104
aggression 9, 30; avoidance of 43; drives 41; and sexual boundary violations 87; and theoretical differences 176
aging: confronting 130; changes in theory and practice 137–142; denial 134–136; developmental model 132; and feeling unseen 129; and neutrality 133; and timelessness 131
Akhtar, Salman 131

aloneness 4, 14, 16–17, 195, 198; capacity to be alone 14, 45–46; and creativity 189, 197; grief 146–147, 154, 156, 164; need for 46; solitary generation 159; termination, after 112, 114; of victims 62, 86; see also loneliness
analytic training 57–58, 118, 169, 181, 183; multiple tracks 174–175; perspectives at beginning of xvii–xviii; rules 105, 118, 141; schisms, impact on 169–172, 179; training analyst 176
antisemitism 161, 181, 186–187
anti-vaxxer 162
Aron, Lew 62, 136, 184, 194, 198
Aronson, Seth 166
attunement 4, 58; autonomy (see agency); disruption of 75; hyper 14–15, 16; illusion of 11, 23, 148; misattunement 12; need for 22
avoidance 24–25, 105, 115–116; of aggression 43; in aging 131–136; attempted 32; of conflict 170, 174; of confrontation 37; due to guilt 83; of dynamics 60, 158; pathologizing 43; of retirement 135; of shame 27; see also sidestepping

baby 148, 195; again xviii, 7; longings 59; metaphor 28; in mother's presence 14; needs 21, 26, 92, 131; patient as 9–10, 23, 45; repair 27; states 21–22, 29, 57; wish 8
balancing 49, 53, 80–81, 163; counterbalancing 201; rebalancing 4, 21, 25–26
Balint, Michael 43, 59
Barron, James 98
Bass, Anthony 21

Baum-Baicker, Cynthia xiv
Beebe, Beatrice 11
being 178; and doing 126, 193, 198–199;
    going on 131, 133, 148, 161; self-states
    60, 195–197; way of 38, 46, 100, 173;
    *see also* doing
Benjamin, Jessica 9–10, 21–22, 184
Berger, Peter 123
Bergmann, Martin 105, 109–110
Bernstein, Jeanne 82
Binswanger, Ludwig 113
Bion, Wilfred 11, 172
bisexuality 193–194
Black Lives Matter 186
*Black Psychoanalysts Speak 186*
borderline patients 7, 139; and sexual
    violations 91
boredom 75–77
boundary 74, 118, 148, 174, 179, 193;
    between analyst and patient 10, 38, 55;
    development of 99, 116; respect for 100;
    rigid xviii; violations (*see* boundary
    violations)
boundary violations: ethical dynamics of
    71; exploitative 75; major 51, 74; post-
    termination 101–102, 110, 117, 119;
    sexual (*see* sexual boundary violations)
bracketing 18, 20, 35, 75, 141; breaches
    (*see* boundary violations; delinquency);
    feeling misunderstood 5; and holding
    12; limits of 54–55, 149, 165 (*see also*
    leaks); mutual 11, 13; reasons for 56;
    while writing 197, 199
Bromberg, Philip 22, 44
Brooklyn College xvii, 88
Buechler, Sandra 166
burnout 79–80, 137

cancer 133
case examples: affect regulation [Mona]
    59–60; aging and reality 140; aging
    [Sam] 129–130; boundaries and
    flexibility 174; buffering shame [Mark]
    23–26; changes and termination
    [Sarah] 63, 99–100, 116–118; cognitive
    impairment 136; Csillag 50; defense
    against grief [Susan and Christie]
    158–159; delinquency [Mr. J] 71, 76–78;
    disavowed needs and delinquency
    [Dr. F, Dr. V] 79–80; foreclosure and
    bracketing [Jonathon] 13; holding
    affect states [Karen] 18–19; holding

and clinician-parents [Samuel] 14–16,
    18, 73–74; holding and dependency 8;
    holding [Margaret Little] 8; leaks in
    holding [Sonia] 54–55; loss and being
    un-held [Tania] 164; non-disclosure
    [Steven] 55–56; post-termination contact
    109–112; reenactment and breaches
    81; resistance [Sally] 34–36, 37–39;
    self-disclosure [John; separation and
    termination [Paul] 108–109; sexual
    boundary violations 86–87, 95–96;
    theory versus practice 177–178;
    tolerating affect [Martha] 16–18
change: and aging 137–142; celebration
    of 113; critique as instrument of
    184–185; in enactments 45; after loss
    154; in post-therapy relationship 111;
    in psychoanalysis (*see* psychoanalysis,
    changes in); and resistance 38–39; in
    therapy 7, 62–63, 109; wish to 40, 49,
    52
character armor 170
classical: critiques of 175; ideal and actual
    177–178; influence on relational ideal
    41–42, 43; missteps in treatment (*see*
    clinical blindness); on mourning
    150–151; perspective of Winnicott 9; and
    resistance 30, 37; training experiences
    141, 173; treatment 7
climate change 162–163, 186
clinical blindness 47, 50
cognitive changes 132–133, 136
Cohen, Leonard 124
collusion 31, 36, 68, 136, 202; with
    boundary violators 94
communism *see* Red Scare
community xiv, 93–94, 95–98, 163–164;
    analytic 75, 85–87, 104–105, 107, 125;
    harm to 91; Jewish 144–150; lack of
    access to 161; and mourning 143; need
    for 68; protecting 94; virtual 167
conflict 109, 111, 123–124, 140–141, 173,
    179; analysis of 9; attachment 60, 115;
    avoidant of 170, 174, 184; dynamics
    47, 166; element 31; mourner's 149;
    needs 81, 202; political 181, 185–187;
    relationships 107; around separation
    192; state 57; about termination 178;
    theoretical 183; unresolved 150–151;
    writers 193
confusion 63; about boundary violations
    86, 91; and clinical theory 177, 183,

190; self 15; about theoretical tribalism
170–171
conscious: containment 11; awareness
78; bracketing 12–13 (*see also*
unconscious, bracketing; unconscious,
disclosure); clinical moment 55;
delinquencies 72–73, 76, 79–80;
of needs 84; shifts in holding 44;
treatment decisions 136
constriction xvii–xviii, 41, 52, 56, 104,
118, 174, 202; of analytic goals 115; of
creative process 192, 199; by disclosure
50; due to aging 118, 132, 138, 141;
of independence 132; legal 92–93; of
neutrality 45; and telehealth 76n2, 164,
167; *see also* refraining
consultation 46, 69, 98, 138, 179
corruption: of behavior and ideal 79–80;
confronting 69; and termination
104–105, 119
countertransference 46, 50, 102, 169,
174; ability to use 58; and adherence to
theory 177–178; coasting in 90, 100;
and delinquency 80; erotic 68, 85, 88;
expressions of 37, 50; negative 49;
normalization of hate 173; resistance
30–31, 39; revisited 42; *see also*
transference
covid 62, 161–167, 183
creativity 125, 202; and aloneness 14;
anxiety (*see* writing, anxieties about);
destruction of 170; potential for 176
critical pluralism 184
criticism 47, 198, 200; critical eye 23,
194; feelings 55; other's work 189;
from parents 16; vulnerability to 190;
Winnicott's 5
critique: adherence 178; allegiance
and 179; anticipation of 190; cross-
theoretical 52, 64, 184–185; danger
of 198; of developmental metaphors
20, 28; evades 191; feminist 10;
relationalist 9, 44, 175; self 42, 51,
181–182, 184, 201; theoretical 180;
vulnerability to 199
Csillag, Veronica 50

Davies, Jody 22
dead third 162; *see also* Gerson,
Samuel
death: aging and 133, 136; of analyst 59;
anxiety 101, 131–132, 139; of child 113;

of Freud 181; inevitability of 137; life
and 101, 125; and mourning
(*see* mourning); unexpected 143; *see
also* mortality
decathexis 101, 150–151, 159; *see also*
classical
delinquency 84; addressing 83; anecdotes
71–72, 76–77; continuum of 74;
definition of 72–73; disavowal of 76;
emotions about 77; inattention 71,
75; relational dynamics 73, 78; and
telehealth 76n2; vulnerability to 75,
79–82; *see also* boundary violations;
sexual boundary violations
denial: of aging 130–131, 133, 135–136,
138; competitive concerns 198; death
147, 154, 159; of dynamics 117; feelings
12; of grief 166–167; guilt and 83;
interpretations of 47; invites 178; of
psychoanalysis' roots 176; unconscious
111; of violations 86, 90–91
dependence 9, 15, 17, 42, 102–104,
107–108; *see also* regression to
dependence
depressed 7, 24, 26, 34, 130
depressive position 68
desire 11, 26, 82, 91, 171–172; analyst's
56n1, 73, 100, 106, 110, 117–118;
balancing 80–81; and creativity 188,
192, 194, 196; Freud's 181; in mourning
158–159; privilege 139; sexual 129; for
vengeance 186
diagnosis: and holding 7, 11, 53; diagnostic
stance 45; psychoanalytic 51
dialectical perspective 3, 183, 189
disclosure 35, 43, 138, 179; decisions about
56, 118; disturbing impact of 47, 50; full
49; inadvertent 54; non 55, 178; polarity
of 20; self 38
disillusionment 68, 80, 89–90, 92, 102,
110–111, 118
dissociation 163; absence of 11, 13;
and bracketing 11–13; contemporary
perspectives 45; due to restraint 50;
dyadic 12; and enactment 41; and
mourning 158; and regression 59; of
relational dynamics 74; and resistance
31; of sexual boundary violations 86;
Winnicott's notions 193
Division 39 Ethics Committee 117,
179
divorce 201

doing 141, 152; anxieties 194–195; being and 126, 193, 198–199; harm caused by 50; issues of 61
doubleness 56–57, 96, 167; of holding 11–12
drive: biological 3; theories 21, 41, 93; *see also* classical
dyad 4, 25, 28, 30, 37, 47–49, 53, 73, 76; dance 11–12; post-termination 103–104, 108, 112, 115; space 13, 16

Eisold, Ken 178
empathic 7, 54, 58, 187; addressing 56, 78; analysis of 9, 46, 49; and boundary violations 51, 94; and breaches 71–74, 81, 85–86; of desires 100, 119; dramatic 39; enactment 5, 19, 53, 108, 144, 174–175; experiences with 173–174; exploration of 43, 47, 116; failure 35–36, 159, 162, 186; holding and 11, 19, 28–29; identifications 140; listener 17, 24–25, 33–34; and mourning 148, 151–152, 154, 167; mutative 41–42; perceived deficits in 169–170; problematic 12; and repair 23, 33, 44–45; and resistance 30–32, 36–38; and restraint 50; "rule breaking" 177–178; and telehealth 76n2; and termination 102, 105, 115; in therapy 14–16, 18, 26, 55, 99; witnessing 163; *see also* responsivity
enfant terrible 202
envy 50; and aging 137; and boundary violations 90, 95; and loss 149; omission of 9; and protégé relationships 104; and termination 119
Epstein, Larry 174
Erikson, Erik xv, 45, 132
Erikson, Joan 132
ethics 202–203; commitment to xvii; committee 117; of post-termination contact 103, 105; transgressions (*see* boundary violations; breaches; delinquency); *see also* morality
excess 52, 162, 199, 201; analyst's expressivity 4; and boundary violations 87–91; correcting 21, 53; examination of 52; openness and 49–50; relational 180; seductive 93; tendency towards 3, 40, 43; *see also* restraint
exculpated 9; honor my 202; ignored 10; memories of 155–156; vision of xviii; *see also* parricide

false self 7; and holding 19, 60; and mourning 147; *see also* Winnicott, Donald
fantasy 22, 68, 90–92, 130, 177, 194; about parents xvii, 10; about patients; sexual 87–88, 93, 129; about therapeutic capacity 27, 60, 63; transference-based 108, 111; about writing 190, 192, 195, 198
father xvii, 13, 88, 136, 157, 192, 194, 196–197; abusive 23–24; death of 143, 146–147, 154, 158
fear 30, 162–163, 192, 194; of annihilation 197; breaking into awareness 139; of causing harm 118; of condemnation 78; denial of 125; of emotions 17; of exposure 126; in family 24; foreclosure 119; of future 137; of losses 4; managing 35, 137; medical crisis 27; and of dying 131; rejection 193; of retaliation 91–92, 180, 190–191, 198; of self states 25; of separating 60; of sexual boundary violations 69; to speak 98; *see also* terror
Feltman, Shirley 174
feminist 129; identification 178; models 175; paternalism 41–42; psychoanalysts 9–10; view of violations 68; writer 42, 192
Fiscalini, John 43
foreclosure: and aging 135, 137; and boundary violations 74, 86, 102; of creativity 192; due to conflict 186; of feelings 140; and grief 149, 158, 165, 167; in post-analytic relationships 115, 119–120; of relational thinking 4, 9, 46; of self-reflectivity 138, 177; in therapy 13, 48, 67, 165, 167
forgetting 108, 134, 136
Fors, Malin 162
Frankel, Jay 82
Freedman, Bert 174
freedom 172; in clinical practice xviii, 43, 55, 139, 178; and delinquencies 76n2, 93; impact of 49; and individuation 115; and loss 112, 135, 147, 150, 167; of mothers 10; of patients 47, 73, 102, 133; in relational analysis 47; from suffering 151
Freudian xviii, 41, 43, 169, 172–173, 175–177; *see also* Freud, Sigmund; supervision 58, 174

Freud, Sigmund 113, 158, 176, 180–181,
    200n6; *see also* classical; Freudian
Friedman, Diane 106
Frommer, Martin 131, 135, 140, 166
Fromm-Reichmann, Frieda xiii

Gabbard, Glen 74, 92
gaps between: baby and adult 45; ideal and
    reality 28, 48, 82, 84, 90, 110, 117, 177,
    201; theory and adaptation 176; theory
    and practice 177–179; virtual and actual
    164–165
generativity 3, 11, 27, 52, 104; in older
    years xv, 132, 137
Gerson, Samuel 162
Ghent, Emmanuel 175
ghost 165; of analytic past 110; ancestors
    138; of sexual boundary violations 85; of
    splits 171, 187; under-mourned 137
gossiping 105; about sexual boundary
    violations 87–89, 93–94
grandiosity 9, 93, 194, 198; *see also*
    narcissism
grandmother 129, 155, 158
Grand, Sue 22, 86, 186
gratification 81, 106, 109, 178; resist
    82; from therapeutic role 80; *see also*
    pleasure
greed 26, 79, 84, 100; *see also* desire;
    selfishness
Guntrip, Harry 4

Hamas 186
Harris, Adrienne 22
hate 18, 49, 150, 172, 186; analytic 53, 84;
    in countertransference 79, 173–174
Hirsch, Irwin 90
Hoffman, Irwin 22, 79
holding-expressivity binary 20–21, 53–54,
    56–57
Holmes Commission 186
Holocaust 27, 62, 181–182, 187
Honig, Richard 98
horror 87–88; of aging and death 132, 136;
    pandemic 161
humor 24–26, 129

idealization 43–44, 45, 109, 132, 151, 172;
    of analysis 28; analyst 10, 41–42, 58,
    84, 96; of autonomy 62; of babyhood 8;
    being 48, 55, 104, 106n1; de-idealizing
    68, 89–90, 92, 96, 98, 110; fantasy 198;
    of holding 11, 58; of motherhood 9,
    82; object 197; and post-termination

friendship 111; preserving 69, 91;
    relationship 107; responsiveness 84;
    self-state 195, 199; separation 115, 159;
    shadow presence of 103; in theoretical
    models 49
ignored: aging 131, 133; analyst 79, 89–90,
    177; the intersubjective 202; other
    orientations 171; patient 24, 33, 35, 37,
    75; the preoedipal father 10; reenactment
    81; roots of psychoanalysis 176; space
    between theory and practice 178;
    termination ideal 117, 119; theoretical
    overlaps 171
immigration 62, 163, 181, 191
impingement 7, 61, 131, 148
impulsivity 46, 117, 177; and lapses 81
inaction 27, 149
infantilization 175
Ingram, Douglas 134–135
inner 4, 15; collapse 188; negotiation and
    delinquencies 81; pressure 79, 195;
    process 148; readiness 5–6; relationships
    99, 102, 151–153; space 16, 126; *see
    also* interiority; internalized
insideness *see* interiority
interiority 4, 14, 18, 165; expand access to
    11, 125, 141, 152; and intersubjectivity
    156; and resistance 38; sustained sense
    of 14–16, 46; tolerance for 16–17, 24,
    34, 196; *see also* inner; internalized
internalized 60, 101, 117, 152, 191; object,
    absent or lost 112, 150–151; object, toxic
    23; relationships 102, 197–198; *see also*
    inner, relationships
interpersonal theory xviii, 9, 31, 180;
    conflict 169–170, 172; influence of
    41–43, 62, 174–175; misuse of theory
    93
interpretation 27–28 47, 134, 139–140;
    as accusation 4; case examples 24, 26,
    34–36, 54; idealization of 58; preclusion
    of 20; premature 5; refraining from 11,
    14, 18–19, 34; rejection of ideas about
    41; replacement of 42; and resistance
    30–32, 34–38; to support holding 7,
    53–54
intimacy 48, 113, 135, 157; avoidance of
    116; wish for 91
invisible 129
Israel 144, 186–187
I-thou 10, 116

Jacobs, Theodore 42–43
James, William 124

Jewish 171, 181–182, 187; family xiii; history 186; holiday 126; holiday 126–127; identified 100; kaddish 146, 153–154, 156; mourning rituals 143–144, 153–154; yizkor 144, 153–157, 159; *see also* antisemitism
Josephs, Lawrence 117
justification 27, 92–93, 116–117, 119, 177; *see also* rationalization
just noticeable difference 173

Kantrowitz, Judy 101, 107–108, 112
Kernberg, Otto 170
Kirsner, Douglas 170
Klein, Melanie 131, 172
Kohut, Heinz 43, 45, 182
Kohut, Thomas 182; *see also* Kohut, Heinz
Kubie, Lawrence 107, 109

Lachmann, Frank 11
Lamm, Maurice 144
lashon hara 94; *see also* gossip
lay analysts 169, 179n2, 182
leaks 12, 20, 36, 54–55, 61
Lehrer, Tom 171
Lester, Eva 74
Levine, Howard 102
limitations 21, 40, 42, 202–203; in ability to be non-disclosing 20, 54–55; acceptance of 132–134; in affect tolerance 17, 25–26, 34; in analytic openness 55–56; in attachment 108; awareness of 63, 136–137; in capacity to change 139; in clinical capacity 39, 67, 80, 84, 168; of contemporary context 20, 62, 167; creativity 199; in holding ability 19, 58; of holding-expressivity binary 53–57; of holding's effectiveness 34–35, 59–61; and idealization (*see* idealization); of mourning rituals 149–150, 165; pandemic 162
listserv 186
Little, Margaret 8; *see also* Winnicott, Donald
Loewald, Hans 21, 43, 85, 109, 151, 172, 175
loneliness 24, 118; *see also* aloneness
loyalty 104, 176, 180, 184

manic defense 130, 132, 162, 195
marriage 99, 116; wedding 153, 155–156
mature 46, 108, 118, 132; adult 21; with age 137, 139–141; decision 90; modes of relating 27, 69, 116, 118

McWilliams, Nancy xviii, 50, 135, 177
mentalization 34–35
mentorship *see* sponsorship
mirror neuron 61
missing tombstones 151
Mitchell, Steven 10, 21, 175, 197
morality xiii, 74, 76, 86; *see also* ethics
mortality 124, 131–132, 135, 157
Moskowitz, Michael 97
mother xvii–xviii, 123, 158, 177–178, 192–193, 195, 201–202; abandonment by 59; absent 24; aging 140; death of 146, 154, 164; depressed 26; good enough 173; memories of 156–157; motherhood 9; presence 14; pulls and pushes of 22; responsive 7–8; similar to 17, 129, 137; subjectivity of 10
mourning: actual loss 143; internalization of object 151; memorialization 152–159; need to 118, 124; processes 102; rituals (*see* mourning rituals); termination 109, 112–115; under-mourned 137
mourning rituals: across cultures 144; reluctant participation 143; shiva 144–150; yizkor 144, 153–157
mutual 118; bracketing 11, 13; capacity for 109; coercion and 103; collusion 136; dyadic dance 12; enactments 177; engagement 4, 14, 17, 64; exchange 49; exploration 20, 42–43, 47; genuinely 108; holding and 54, 57, 167; knowing 111; move towards 141; mutuality 21, 23, 28–29, 41, 53, 56, 156; post-termination relationships 69, 110, 116; recognition 10; regulation 22; relationship 9; resistance 31, 106; respect 184–185, 187

*Nakba* 187
narcissism: holding 18, 23; injury 129; patients 149; of small differences 176; vulnerability 194
Nass, Martin 135
negation 80, 98, 118, 130, 140; without 147, 156, 167; of capacity 134; of our experience 12; of reality 133; of sensitivity 34; of subjectivity 10, 74; theoretical differences 64, 184; by traditional psychoanalysis 175; and writing 189–190
nepotism 69, 104
neurotic patients 7
neutrality 41, 45, 49, 133, 177–178
nostalgia 155–156, 158

not me 86
NYU Postdoc 169–170, 174–175, 180, 182

object 7, 10, 26, 190; bad 9, 45; external
    10 (*see also* other); fantasies 194; good
    60; internalized 23, 112, 150–151; lost
    112, 150, 159; love 157, 159; new 23,
    109; old 14, 101, 156; parental 62, 195;
    selfobject failure 12, 19; threatening
    196–197, 199; usage xviii, 53, 156; *see
    also* object relations theory
objectification 129
object relations theory: conflict with other
    theories 43, 172; experiences with 58,
    141, 173–176; influence on relational
    theorists 41–44
October 7 attacks 186
oedipal 192, 194, 197; *see also* classical;
    Freud, Sigmund
Ogden, Thomas 22, 81; *see also* reverie
omnipotent: analyst 9, 41, 68; denial 135;
    fantasies 194; parents' 16
other 34–37, 73, 94, 103, 127, 167; analytic
    114; bonds to 163; boundaries against
    38; centeredness 68; communication to
    189, 199; destructiveness towards 161;
    engagement with 53–54, 187, 190, 192,
    194; experience of 116; focus on 119;
    hatred of 186; idealized 90; lost 165;
    mother as 10, 22; need for 153; othering
    31; otherness 11, 13–14; psychoanalytic
    40, 51, 52, 64, 170–172, 175, 182–185;
    responsibility for 135; self and 47, 115,
    126; to share with 93; soothing 16;
    specter of 188; threatening 197; using
    148; validating 17; worry about 198

Palestinian 186–187
parricide 175, 187, 192
participant 25, 43, 90, 156
participation 32, 35–37, 43, 47, 63, 73; in
    boundary violations 98; in bracketing 20;
    in commemorative rituals 167; passive
    90; in remembering 152
Pfeffer, Arnold 109
phobic response 158; *see also* avoidance
Pizer, Barbara 98
pleasing others 15, 47, 172
pleasure: block 158; and caution 100; and
    desire 106; of feeling special 93; of
    gossiping 88; of idealization 48, 104;

of post-termination contact 110–111;
    prurient 87; seeking 41; stolen 81;
    *see also* gratification
pluralism 125–126, 181, 183–185
polarization 20–21, 126; conflict 123–124;
    dichotomy 3; of dyad 30; earlier 52;
    moving past 184, 201; in psychoanalytic
    community 125, 180; tendency towards
    40
police 161, 163; analytic 117; moral 76
post-termination contact 69, 99–101 112,
    120; dynamics 115; and ideal 102, 105;
    mentorship 103–104; motivation for
    103, 106–107, 115, 117–118; moving
    beyond transference 108–109, 116; risks
    110–111, 119
Powell, Dionne 186
prayer 146, 154–156
pregnancy xviii, 13
Prince, Robert 181
privacy 14, 18, 190–193; need for 4, 20, 46,
    48–49, 55–56
protege *see* sponsorship
psychic 102; capacities 125; elements 85;
    intrapsychic 152; mind 92; space 161
psychoanalytic sequel *see* post-termination
    contact
psychotic patients 7
pulls and pushes 22, 67
Putin, Vladimir 163

racism 186
rationalization 106, 117, 119; as breach
    76; delinquencies 79–80, 83; violations
    90–93; of withholding 27; *see also*
    justification
rebelling 58, 173; against earlier theories
    43, 52; and misdemeanors 80, 82;
    *see also* constriction
recognition 15, 131, 184, 186; need for
    28; nonrecognition 27, 34; resistance
    to 35; resonant 12; shared 77; of
    subjectivity 7
Red Scare xvii
refraining 50, 54; mourning, during 145–146;
    from naming sexual transgressors 94n2; in
    therapy 15, 19, 34, 36
refugee 62, 163
regression to dependence: in therapy
    7; case examples of 59–60, 63; in
    contemporary work 19; and holding 14;

original meaning of 27; and repair
(*see* repair); risks of 59–62, 141;
Winnicott's vision of xviii, 8, 43–44, 58
Reich, Annie 109; *see also* character
armor
relational theory 44–50; self-examination
of 52–53; of telehealth 61; of theoretical
models 43–44, 57, 185; in training
approaches 56–57; of virtual interactions
165; *see also* aging; denial
religious 114; institutions 171; Judaism
(*see* Jewish); rituals (*see* mourning
rituals)
relinquishment 101; of analytic occupation
36; of analytic relationship 105–109,
152; of authority 47; and loss 113; object
151; of past 151
Renik, Owen 101–102
repair 35–36, 97–99, 140–141, 164, 201;
analyst's capacity to 42, 142; the baby
27, 45; enacted 22, 33, 45, 51; fantasy
22; gradual 39; maternal (analytic)
xviii, 7, 9, 62; real 8; relational 58, 158;
rupture and 184; symbolic 38
repeated: relationship 7, 9, 79; experience
32, 59; remembering 151; *see also*
repetition compulsion
repetition compulsion 187
resiliency 17, 19, 48, 61, 116, 137, 141;
limitations of 167
responsivity 16, 22, 26, 84; and clinical
theory 177, 178; and creativity 196, 199;
and loss 167; in relational analysts 43,
67; Winnicott's vision of xviii, 7
restraint: analytic 51; downsides 50; and
expressivity (*see* restraint- expressivity
continuum); and holding 53; unintended
55
restraint-expressivity continuum 21, 54
retirement 134–137
reverie 75, 81, 83
rigid 63, 82, 98, 117, 199; aging 118;
boundaries of shiva 148; boundaries
xviii; defenses 36; Freudian 169,
173–174; position 74; principles 40,
52; and regret 64; training 56, 132, 135,
137–138; *see also* constriction
rupture 99, 111, 184

Salberg, Jill 101
Sandler, Joseph 11, 26, 43, 176–177

satisfaction 48, 99, 116, 135; of personal
needs 72, 77, 81, 100; self 67; *see also*
gratification
Schacter, Joseph 102, 107
schizoid 7; detachment 158; paranoid-
schizoid 186
Schore, Allan 44; *see also* mirror neuron
Schwartz, Murray 181
self-analysis 25, 102
self-consciousness 15, 25, 93
self-holding 19, 60; *see also* Winnicott,
Donald
self-indulgence 119, 138
selfishness 80, 84, 135; *see also* greed
selfobject 43–44; failure 12, 19; *see also*
Kohut, Heinz
self-reflectivity 24, 53, 99, 111; of analyst
48, 58, 90, 138, 176; on boundary
violations 95; capacity for 28–29, 116
Seligman, Stephen 45
sensitivity xiv, 4, 8, 16, 34, 60, 71, 91, 116;
insensitivity 140
separate 22, 54, 108, 193, 195; connected
and 157, 159; difficult patient 4; from
dyad 4, 38; members 179; move toward
102; need to 107; perspectives 192;
sense of being 115–116; separation-
individuation 107–108; tolerance of 11,
14, 55, 67; unable to 153; wish to 173;
from world 144
sexual boundary violations 67–68, 100;
consequences of naming offenders
94–96; decision to report 87–92;
enactments as 51; gossip about 93–94;
historical 85; justification 92–93;
personal encounters with 86–87, 95–96;
restorative justice 97–98
shadow 12–13, 22, 115–116; of mortality
135; presence 103; traumatic 88; of
violations 85
shame 4, 33, 42; and boundary violations
86, 88–89; and delinquencies 77, 80;
denial or disavowal of 95, 97, 125;
formulations of 30; in therapy 23–28, 59
Sheehi, Lara 186
sidestepping 47, 58, 119, 178, 194; in aging
131–132, 134; due to idealization 115;
judgment 76; and misdemeanors 83;
negative transference-countertransference
49; response to sexual breach 88; worries
198; *see also* avoidance

siege mentality 170
socialism *see* Red Scare
splitting: in field 64, 169–171, 179–181, 185n4, 186–187
sponsorship 103–104; *see also* post-termination contact
Stein, Ruth 18
Sternberg, Robert xiv
Stern, Donnell 22
Stine, John 134–135
suicide 63 158
Sullivan, Harry 41, 43, 75
superego 83, 106, 118–119, 141
symbolic 3, 88, 187, 192, 196; aliveness 25–26; capacity for 32, 34; embodied 73; hatred 79, 84; mourning 144–146, 151, 157; parent xviii, 7, 197; post-termination 103–104, 114; repair 7, 38; repetition 59; sibling 13, 191

tension 49, 82, 87, 132, 134, 199; between holding and mutuality 54; between interior and intersubjective 156; between recognition and non-recognition 189; between theories 175
termination 25, 106, 109, 111–114, 120, 152; abrupt 37; failing to 102; memorializing 153, 157; postponed 105; post- termination contact (*see* post-termination contact); setting date 99, 101; therapeutic impact 101–102; traumatic 108; vision of 107
terror 123, 162, 181, 191; of abandonment 54; control 188; of loss 158; of mortality 125, 133, 135; of pandemic 163; *see also* fear
Thoreau, Henry 6
threat 86, 88, 158, 167, 199–200; of aging 137; of annihilation 125, 131, 191; contemporary 187, 190; of covid 162–163, 165; exclusion of 193–194, 196–197; of exposure 26; ideals 98; legal 79; to patient 31, 33; to post-termination contact 111, 117; to self-esteem 76; sense of intactness 59; of theoretical schisms 170–171, 180, 182–183, 185
timelessness 131, 138–139, 152–153
transference 101–102, 106, 138, 174; exploration 16; listening for 129; love 105; negative 49; parental 118; and real relationships 103; resolved 109, 111, 116; unresolved 108, 110; *see also* countertransference

transitional: object 27; space 27, 159, 193–194, 200; transitionality xviii, 173
trauma 16, 22, 41, 50, 98, 100, 131; and aging 124; and Covid 125; early 7, 59, 99, 108, 112, 141; and frame 174; history 24–25, 34, 116–117; modern-day 161–163, 187; and mourning 112–113, 146, 149–152, 154, 156–158, 165; relational 7, 45; and resistance 32; and sexual boundary violations 85–89, 92–93, 95–96; and splits in psychoanalysis 181–182; and witnessing 27, 36; *see also* Holocaust
true self 7–8; *see also* false self; Winnicott, Donald
*The Truman Show* 123–124
Trump, Donald 162
twinship 13

Ukraine 161n1, 163
unanalyzable 102, 106
unconscious: bracketing 12–13, 20; changes in aging 139; changes in mutuality 29; collective 94; collusion 31; communication 73, 77; disclosure 49, 54, 56; enactments 81; evasion of affect 30, 32; identifications 172–173; inattention 83; influences on 194–195, 197; informed by 44, 55, 201; intersection of 42; limiting factors 19; motivations after boundary violations 80–81, 96; parental interpretation of xvii; and post-termination relationships 104, 107, 111, 118; self-restoration 75; sensibilities 69; undoing 36, 110, 201; and writer's block 190–192

validation 15, 32, 34, 104
Viorst, Judith 106
vulnerability 33–34, 64, 83, 117, 119, 140–141; acknowledgment of 124–125; adapt to 177; and aging 133–134, 136, 139; and boundary violations 51, 74–75, 82, 90–91, 96; to caricature 4; counter 194–195; to criticism 190–192, 199; emotional 44, 131; feelings of 17; and mourning 166–167; to retaliation 88, 92; to self-doubt 192; self-states 45; shame 23, 26, 28; of theory 40, 47–49

waiting 8, 13; as clinical technique 15, 25, 49; in shiva 147
Wallerstein, Robert 170

want *see* wish
Warshaw, Susan 22
Weber, Ernst 173n1
wedding *see* marriage
Whitebook, Joel 181
Willock, Brent 172
Wilson, Mitchell 106
Winnicott, Donald 12–14, 18, 59, 131, 136; critiques of 9; on defensive function 60–61; experiences with 5; on hatred 84; influence on others 174; influence on Slochower xiv, 64, 173, 175, 197; on maternal holding 3–4, 8; on maternal repair 7; on parenting xvii-xviii; on regression 19, 43; on schisms 180; sensibility 6; on subjectivity 53; on termination 120; *see also* Winnicottian
Winnicottian: being 161, 193; identification 173, 175, 179; model 82; thinking 175, 201
wish 18–19, 34–35, 55–56, 61–62, 67, 77, 171–172, 174–175; analyst and patient's 21, 48; baby 8; for change 39; conscious 13; to cross boundaries 88; family 143; for freedom xviii; guilt about 87; to heal 28, 99, 138, 140; for mourning rituals 153, 155, 164; and need 9; pathologizes 46; post-termination 69, 100–103, 106–107, 114–120; for privacy 20, 47–49; professional 40, 52; to protect 13, 88–89, 91; to reassure 133; and regret 64; to retire 134–135; set aside 17–18, 82; for time alone 63, 149
witnessing 17, 23, 25, 38, 126, 168; activism/enacted 163; boundary violations/indirect 85–86; experience of 95, 98; lack of 86; mourning 148, 152, 156, 165, 167; psychoanalytic ritual xvii, 68; and sociopolitical differences 161–162; termination as loss of 114–115; therapeutic power of 27; and victim 96; virtual 164
writing: anxieties about 190–200; attempts at 188; disavowal 95; early relational 21, 44; feeling exposed 196; and gender 192–193; memoir 157; and memory 156; process of xiv; as relational act 189–190

Yanof, Judith 102
Young-Bruehl, Elizabeth 181

Zionism 186

For Product Safety Concerns and Information please contact our EU
representative  GPSR@taylorandfrancis.com
Taylor & Francis Verlag GmbH, Kaufingerstraße 24, 80331 München, Germany

www.ingramcontent.com/pod-product-compliance
Lightning Source LLC
Chambersburg PA
CBHW050640280326
41932CB00015B/2717

9 781032 691527